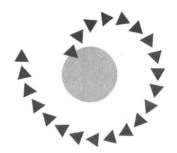

Recent Advances in
SURGERY
37

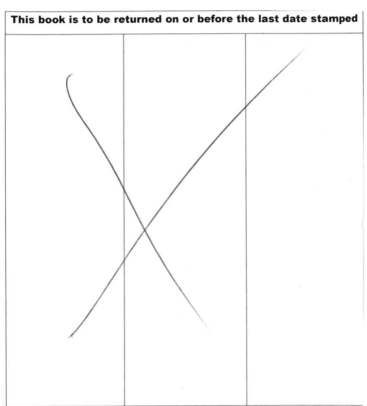

Recent Advances in
SURGERY
37

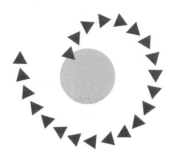

Editor

Irving Taylor MD ChM FRCS FMedSci FHEA
Professor of Surgery and Vice Dean
UCL Medical School
University College London
London, UK

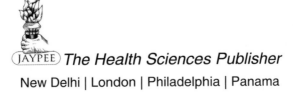

The Health Sciences Publisher

New Delhi | London | Philadelphia | Panama

Jaypee Brothers Medical Publishers (P) Ltd

Headquarters
Jaypee Brothers Medical Publishers (P) Ltd.
4838/24, Ansari Road, Daryaganj
New Delhi 110 002, India
Phone: +91-11-43574357
Fax: +91-11-43574314
E-mail: jaypee@jaypeebrothers.com

Overseas Offices

J.P. Medical Ltd.
83, Victoria Street, London
SW1H 0HW (UK)
Phone: +44-20 3170 8910
Fax: +44(0)20 3008 6180
E-mail: info@jpmedpub.com

Jaypee Medical Inc.
The Bourse
111, South Independence Mall East
Suite 835
Philadelphia, PA 19106, USA
Phone: +1 267-519-9789
E-mail: jpmed.us@gmail.com

Jaypee Brothers Medical Publishers (P) Ltd.
Bhotahity, Kathmandu, Nepal
Phone: +977-9741283608
E-mail: kathmandu@jaypeebrothers.com

Jaypee-Highlights Medical Publishers Inc.
City of Knowledge, Bld. 237, Clayton
Panama City, Panama
Phone: +1 507-301-0496
Fax: +1 507-301-0499
E-mail: cservice@jphmedical.com

Jaypee Brothers Medical Publishers (P) Ltd.
17/1-B, Babar Road, Block-B, Shaymali
Mohammadpur, Dhaka-1207
Bangladesh
Mobile: +08801912003485
E-mail: jaypeedhaka@gmail.com

Website: www.jaypeebrothers.com
Website: www.jaypeedigital.com

Inquiries for bulk sales may be solicited at: jaypee@jaypeebrothers.com

Recent Advances in Surgery—37

First Edition: **2015**

ISBN: 978-93-5152-698-8

Printed at: Samrat Offset Pvt. Ltd.

Contributors

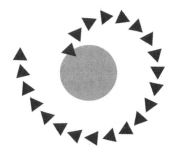

Akshay Anand Agarwal MS
Senior Resident
Department of General Surgery
King George's Medical University
Lucknow, Uttar Pradesh, India

Manit Arya MD FRCS
Senior Lecturer and Hon Consultant
Urology, University College Hospital
London, UK and The Barts Cancer
Institute, Queen Mary University of
London, UK

Giles Bond-Smith MBBS BSc FRCS
Senior Clinical Fellow
HPB and Liver Transplant Unit
Royal Free Hospital
London, UK

Clarisa Choh FRCS
Specialist Registrar
University Hospital Southampton
Southampton, UK

David Cunningham MD FRCP FmedSci
Consultant Medical Oncologist
Department of Gastrointestinal
Oncology
The Royal Marsden Hospital
London, UK

Khaled Dawas MA MD FRCS (Gen)
Senior Lecturer and Consultant
Oesophago-gastric Surgeon
University College London
Division of Surgery and
Interventional Science
London, UK

Thomas Dudding MD FRCS
Consultant Colorectal and Pelvic
Floor Surgeon
University Hospital Southampton
Southampton, UK

Daren Francis MD FRCS
Consultant Colorectal Surgeon
Barnet and Chase Farm Hospital
London, UK

Giuseppe Kito Fusai MS FRCS
Consultant HPB Surgeon
Royal Free Hospital
London, UK

Gareth Griffiths MB ChB MD FRCS(Ed)
FRCS(Eng)
Chairman of the SAC in
General Surgery
Consultant Vascular Surgeon
Ninewells Hospital
Dundee, UK

Vimal Hariharan FRCS
John Radcliffe Hospital
Oxford
UK

Shameen Jaunoo BSc(Hons) MBBS
ChM FRCS
Post CCT Fellow in
Oesophago-gastric Surgery
University Hospital, Coventry, UK

Nicholas Jenkins BM BSc FRCA
Anaesthetic Registrar
Queen Alexandra Hospital
Portsmouth, UK

John D Kelly MD FRCS
Professor of Urology
University College Hospital
London, UK

Jitendra Kumar Kushwaha MS FLCS
Assistant Professor
Department of General Surgery
King George's Medical University
Lucknow, Uttar Pradesh, India

Adam M Lewis CVO FRCS
Past Programme Director CORESS

Satvinder Mudan FRCS BSc MD
Consultant Surgeon
Division of Surgery and Cancer
Imperial College, London
Academic Department of Surgery
The Royal Marsden Hospital
London, UK

Samrat Mukherjee MS MRCS
Specialist Trainee in General Surgery
London Deanery, UK

Rowan W Parks MB BCh BAO MD FRCSI
                FRCS(Ed) FFST(Ed)
Professor of Surgical Sciences and
Honorary Consultant Surgeon
University of Edinburgh
Royal Infirmary of Edinburgh
Edinburgh, UK

Siân Pugh BM (Hons) BSc MRCS
Clinical Research Fellow
General Surgery University
Surgery University of Southampton
Southampton, UK

Toby Richards MD FRCS
Senior Lecturer and Honorary
Consultant in Vascular Surgery,
University College London Hospitals
NHS Foundation Trust

Andrew J Robson MA BM BCh MRCS
Specialty Registrar in General Surgery
Royal Infirmary of Edinburgh
Edinburgh, UK

Taimur Shah FRCS
Specialist Registrar and Clinical
Research Fellow Urology, University
College Hospital
London, UK

Arifa Siddika MBBS FRCS
Registrar Colorectal Surgery
Broomfield Hospital, Chelmsford
Essex, UK

Shahab Siddiqui BSc MD FRCS
Consultant Colorectal Surgeon
Broomfield Hospital, Chelmsford
Essex, UK

Kul Ranjan Singh MS MCh
Assistant Professor
Department of General Surgery
King George's Medical University
Lucknow, Uttar Pradesh, India

Saumya Singh MS
Senior Resident
Department of General Surgery
King George's Medical University
Lucknow, Uttar Pradesh, India

S Sinha FRCS
Specialist Registrar in
General Surgery
NE Thames Rotation
London Deanery, UK

Alistair AP Slesser MBBS (Lond)
                MRCS (Eng) MSc DIC
Clinical Research Fellow
Division of Surgery and Cancer
Imperial College
London, UK

Frank CT Smith BSc MD FRCS FEBVS FHEA
Professor of Vascular Surgery and
Surgical Education
University of Bristol, UK
Programme Director, Confidential
Reporting System for Surgery
(CORESS)

Elizabeth Smyth MB BCh Msc
Clinical Research Fellow
Department of Gastrointestinal
Oncology
The Royal Marsden Hospital
London, UK

Abhinav Arun Sonkar MS FACS FUICC
FRCS (Eng) (Corresponding author)
Professor and Head
Department of General Surgery
King George's
Medical University
Lucknow, Uttar Pradesh, India

Mike Stroud OBE FRCS
Consultant Gastroenterologist
Southampton, UK

Lt Col Nigel Tai FRCS
Department of Vascular and Trauma
Royal London Hospital, London, UK

Claire Warden FRCS
Consultant Colorectal Surgeon
Groote Schuur Hospital
Cape Town, South Africa

Miss C Webster MBChB MRCS RAF
Specialist Registrar
Department of Vascular Surgery and
Trauma, Royal London Hospital
London, UK

Denis C Wilkins MD FRCS
Past President, Association of
Surgeons, Great Britain and Ireland

Preface

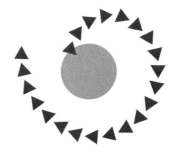

In this volume of Recent Advances in Surgery, I have attempted to include topics in which there have been recent major changes involving patient care. Each subject has been written by experts in the field and provides an up-to-date review designed to be of value to surgeons taking professional examinations in General Surgery. I also hope that the issues covered will be of practical interest to all surgeons wishing to keep abreast of changes within the broad field of General Surgery.

The general themes include a review of modern day surgical training, the importance of confidential reporting systems in surgical practice, an update on the use of intravenous fluids and the important issue of the management of knife injuries.

Concepts relating to gastrointestinal surgery include the management of gastric cancer, gastroesophageal reflux, resectability in pancreatic cancer, management of synchronous colorectal liver metastases, enhanced recovery following colorectal resection, the use of robotics, and anal fistula management. Other specialist topics include modern prostate cancer management, phyllodes tumour of the breast, the management of varicose veins and superficial venous incompetence. The volume concludes with a review of recent randomised controlled trials in surgery.

I hope readers agree that this volume maintains the high standards of previous editions. I am most grateful to all our contributors for taking the time to provide comprehensive reviews of each topic.

Irving Taylor

Acknowledgements

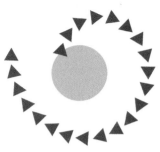

We are grateful to the staff of M/s Jaypee Brothers Medical Publishers (P) Ltd, New Delhi, India, and Ms Ritika Verma (Development Editor) in particular for expert assistance in the production of the book.

Contents

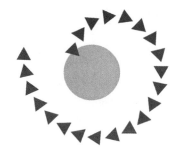

Section 1: Surgery in General

1. **What's New in Surgical Training**   **3**
   Andrew J Robson, Gareth Griffiths, Rowan W Parks
   - Curricula in Surgical Training   *3*
   - Assessment in Surgical Training   *5*
   - Selection into Surgical Specialties   *7*
   - Surgical Training within Modern Working Regulations   *10*
   - The Applicability of Surgical Simulation and Courses   *11*

2. **Confidential Reporting Systems in Surgical Practice**   **15**
   Frank CT Smith, Adam M Lewis, Denis C Wilkins
   - Confidential Reporting: Lessons from Aviation   *15*
   - The Confidential Reporting System for Surgery   *16*
   - National Confidential Enquiry into Patient Outcomes
     and Deaths (NCEPOD)   *19*
   - The NPSA and the NRLS   *21*

3. **The Management of Knife Injuries**   **25**
   Miss C Webster, Lt Col Nigel Tai
   - Philosophy of Approach   *25*
   - Immediate Assessment and Investigation   *27*
   - Investigation   *30*
   - Resuscitation   *30*
   - Management   *33*
   - Injury Prevention   *33*

4. **An Update on Intravenous Fluids in Surgical Practice**   **38**
   Mike Stroud
   - Problems of Prescribing IV Fluids in Surgery   *38*
   - Assessment of IV Fluid and Electrolyte Needs in
     Surgical Patients   *42*
   - Reassessment and Monitoring   *45*
   - Choice of IV Fluid Type   *45*

Section 2: Upper GI Surgery

5. **Recent Concept in the Management of Gastric Cancer**   55
Shameen Jaunoo

- Classification of Gastric Cancer   55
- Clinical Manifestations, Diagnosis and Staging   57
- Treatment   58

6. **Surgical Aspects of Gastro-oesophageal Reflux**   72
Samrat Mukherjee, Khaled Dawas

- Initial Management   73
- Investigations   73
- Surgical Management   75
- Endoscopic Procedures   82
- Newer Procedures   83

7. **Determining Resectability in Pancreatic Cancer**   87
Giles Bond-Smith, Giuseppe Kito Fusai

- Definitions   87
- Increasing Resectability Rates   91

Section 3: Lower GI Surgery

8. **Enhanced Recovery Following Colorectal Resection**   101
Vimal Hariharan, Daren Francis

- Special Considerations   105

9. **Management of Fistula-in-ano**   108
Clarisa Choh, Claire Warden, Thomas Dudding

- Pathogenesis   108
- Diagnosis   108
- Imaging   109
- Classification   110
- Initial Treatment   110
- Advanced Treatments   111
- Filling the Tract   112
- Ligation of the Tract   115
- Obliteration of the Tract   116

10. **The Use of Robotics in Colorectal Surgery**   120
Arifa Siddika, Shahab Siddiqui

- History of Robotic Surgery   120
- Robotic Surgery—Advantages and Disadvantages   120
- Colorectal Surgery   123

- Surgery for Internal and External Rectal Prolapse   *126*
- Future Developments   *126*

Section 4: Surgical Oncology

11. Modern Prostate Cancer Management   **131**
Taimur Shah, Manit Arya, John D Kelly

- Screening   *131*
- Diagnosis   *132*
- Treatment   *135*
- Metastatic Disease   *140*

12. Phyllodes Tumour of Breast: Still a Challenge   **147**
Abhinav Arun Sonkar, Akshay Anand Agarwal, Kul Ranjan Singh,
Saumya Singh, Jitendra Kumar Kushwaha

- Clinical Presentation   *147*
- Role of Preoperative Investigations   *148*
- Management   *152*

13. Management of Patients with Primary Colorectal
Cancer and Synchronous Liver Metastasis   **160**
Alistair AP Slesser, Elizabeth Smyth, David Cunningham,
Satvinder Mudan

- Selection for Surgery   *161*
- Oncological Management   *163*
- Operative Planning   *164*
- Discussion   *166*
- Irresectable Synchronous Colorectal Liver Metastases   *167*
- Adjunctive Treatments   *168*
- Extra-Hepatic Metastases   *168*
- Follow-Up   *169*

Section 5: Vascular

14. Superficial Venous Incompetence and
Varicose Vein Management   **175**
S Sinha, Toby Richards

- Role of Preoperative Duplex Ultrasound Scanning (USS)   *177*
- Surgical and Closure Techniques   *177*
- Efficacy and Cost-Effectiveness of Endovenous Techniques   *181*
- Venous Ulceration   *181*
- Compression Hosiery   *183*
- Recurrence and Pelvic Vein Reflux   *184*

Section 6: Clinical Trials

15. **A Review of Recent Randomised Controlled Trials in Surgery**   **193**
    Siân Pugh, Nicholas Jenkins
    - Oesophagogastric   *193*
    - Hepatopancreatobiliary   *194*
    - Colorectal   *197*
    - Breast   *199*

    Index   *203*

Section
1

Surgery in General

1

Chapter

What's New in Surgical Training

Andrew J Robson, Gareth Griffiths, Rowan W Parks

INTRODUCTION

Many aspects of postgraduate surgical training in the United Kingdom have changed significantly over the past decade. Some of these were precipitated by the Modernising Medical Careers (MMC) initiative, but others have been due to changes in European Working Time Regulations (EWTR) and General Medical Council (GMC) regulatory developments. This chapter will consider the evolution of defined curricula and assessment, development of selection methodology, training within modern working regulations and the applicability of surgical simulation and courses.

CURRICULA IN SURGICAL TRAINING

The concept of a curriculum to guide learning arose in Ancient Greece and its modern format was defined in the 20th century.[1] Educational theory suggests several aspects to comprise a curriculum:

- Definition of the required endproduct, planning training to deliver this and testing trainees to ensure the objectives have been met.
- The process of interaction between trainers and trainees and how knowledge is shared.
- The detailed list of knowledge and skills required (syllabus).
- Development of the required set of adjunctive behaviours and values.
- The testing strategy.

This approach provides a useful framework on which to base the design of a training programme. The most recent version of the UK General Surgery curriculum will be used as an example.

For most of the 500 years of formal surgical training, the "curriculum" essentially equated to the body of surgical knowledge that existed. Individual practitioners taught their own particular skills to their apprentices. Surgery only evolved into the specialties we know today during the 20th century as technological advances allowed more specialised practice to develop. During this time, the "curriculum" came to be described in terms of the contents of standard texts on the specialties.

The first attempts at creating a curriculum took place around 2001 when a 12-page General Surgery curriculum was published. This briefly described training programmes and discussed the concept of a general surgeon as being one who could manage an emergency take, was capable of independent practice in general surgery, was trained to an advanced level in one or more sub-specialties within general surgery, and would be able to move between sub-specialties as a consultant.

Following a review of postgraduate medical education, MMC was introduced in 2007. One of the provisions was that all postgraduate medical training should be guided by defined curricula. In response, the Royal Colleges of Surgery established the Intercollegiate Surgical Curriculum Project (subsequently renamed the Intercollegiate Surgical Curriculum Programme—ISCP) and introduced formal curricula to meet GMC standards. The 2007 General Surgery curriculum and its later revisions detail the knowledge, clinical and technical skills required to complete training. An updated 2010 version added more detail on adjuvant skills and behaviours (leadership, judgement and professionalism), emphasised progressive skill acquisition and provided improved clarity.

Within the United Kingdom, the GMC is responsible for regulating all medical training and currently recognises 10 surgical specialties (Cardiothoracic Surgery, General Surgery, Neurosurgery, Oral and Maxillofacial Surgery, Otorhinolaryngology, Paediatric Surgery, Plastic and Reconstructive Surgery, Trauma and Orthopaedic Surgery, Urology, Vascular Surgery) and one sub-specialty (Paediatric Cardiac Surgery). Whilst many of the surgical specialities have special interest areas, it should be noted that the GMC have no formal register of these.

The most recent revision of the General Surgery curriculum (2013)[2] lists a specified number of special interest areas, but there are many more commonly discussed as having sub-specialty or even specialty status (Table 1.1).

Although it is recognised that the clinical development of these special interest areas has improved patient care and outcomes, the unintended consequence has been a reduced interest in the generality of emergency general surgery care. Trainees and consultants whose special interest lies outside the gastrointestinal tract have felt increasingly unable to provide emergency general surgery care, the great majority of which involves abdominal or gastrointestinal pathology. Some hospitals have attempted to address this by appointing emergency care surgeons, but this model is not universally supported and there are concerns regarding the long-term career development of surgeons in such posts. These challenges are not unique to surgical specialties, and the recent Shape of Training Review led by Professor David Greenaway has recognised this and proposed a further reform of postgraduate education and training with a greater emphasis on training in the general area of broad specialities with the potential to credential in an area of specialisation.[3]

Table 1.1: General surgery curriculum (2013)		
GMC recognised	*2013 curriculum recognised "special interest areas"*	*Other popularly described interest areas***
General surgery	Upper gastrointestinal (GI) surgery	Oesophagogastric
	Colorectal surgery	Bariatric
	Breast surgery	Benign upper GI
	Transplant Surgery	Hepatopancreatobiliary
	Endocrine Surgery	Hepatobiliary
		Pancreatic
	General surgery of childhood*	Pelvic floor surgery
	Advanced trauma surgery*	Functional colorectal surgery
	Remote and rural surgery*	Emergency surgery

*May only be developed under the 2013 curriculum alongside one of the main special interests.
**This list is not exhaustive.

The 2013 General Surgery curriculum is explicit that trainees must develop skills required for independent practice in emergency general surgery. They should also start to develop a special interest (as listed above), but the level of skill required in complex or uncommon procedures has been amended to recognise that it is not possible to train to a level required for independent practice in such conditions within the time allocated whilst also developing adequate emergency general surgery skills. Knowledge and skill levels are now clearly set for each component of general surgery for all trainees regardless of their special interest.

Key Points

- Surgical curricula should include a clear syllabus, encourage professional behaviours, employ appropriate assessment methodology and guide training to produce the desired standard of graduates from the programme.
- Surgical specialisation is a relatively recent phenomenon, which has improved patient care but reduced the commitment to emergency general surgery. The Shape of Training Review has recommended a greater emphasis on training across a more general specialty area.
- The UK surgical curricula define knowledge, clinical skills and technical skills that are assessed by a combination of formal examinations and work-based assessments.

ASSESSMENT IN SURGICAL TRAINING

Assessment is integral to a curriculum and is undergoing revision within surgery, partly in response to the changes described above and partly because of the development of methodology of assessment systems. In principle, design and content of assessments are dictated by the curriculum and should test abilities appropriately and transparently.

The three main areas requiring assessment are knowledge, clinical skills and technical skills. Knowledge is assessed in Intercollegiate examinations that lead to a Fellowship of one of the Royal Colleges of Surgeons (FRCS). The design and content of the examination are changing to map to the new curriculum with equal emphasis within all sections on emergency general surgery and on the trainee's special interest. The utility, reliability and validity of clinical and oral examinations have been questioned, but it is a widely held view within the surgical community that these formats are important to emulate everyday clinical discussions and to evaluate a trainee's ability to reason and apply sound judgement in decision making. This is what gives the FRCS its high level of face validity. Recognising the need for reliability, structured questions and guidance notes for examiners provide a framework on which to assess each trainee as uniformly as possible and the quality assurance of the whole process is rigorous.

Clinical and technical skills are largely tested in the workplace, although the FRCS examination does also test clinical skills. Workplace-based assessments (WBAs) are divided into case-based discussions (CBDs), clinical encounters (CEXs), direct observation of procedural skills (DOPSs), procedure-based assessments (PBAs) and Multi-Source Feedback (MSF).[4] CBDs and CEXs test clinical skills, DOPSs assess simple procedures whilst PBAs test operative technical skills. Trainees are required to undertake a minimum of 40 assessments yearly to demonstrate engagement with training and provide a record of progressive acquisition of skills. Validity of the assessments is enhanced by ensuring each is performed by three or more assessors. The 2013 curriculum requires trainees to build a portfolio of WBAs demonstrating clinical skills in all the components of general surgery (emergency, special interest, and nonspecial interest) and technical skills in emergency surgery and in their special interest.

There is increasing appreciation of the difference between formative assessment (informal, to indicate progress and highlight areas needing development) and summative assessment (formal, to determine achievement as measured against the curriculum). Current WBAs are used interchangeably and there can be confusion as to their true purpose. There is a suggestion, currently being piloted, that WBAs be divided into supervised learning events and assessments of performance. The type of assessment, i.e. CBD or PBA, may not change but the usage and detail of their scoring system would alter to reflect their application in a formative or summative capacity.

The 2013 curriculum is more specific than before in requiring logbook evidence of the breadth of operative experience. Target experience (numbers of cases) has been set at a relatively low level and corresponds to the first quartile of a group of recently successful graduates awarded their Certificate of Completion of Training (CCT). The curriculum also requires defined evidence of achievement in research publications and presentations, audit and quality improvement, teaching, management skills, courses and conferences attended. The curriculum details requirements for professional skills, nonoperative technical skills and health promotion—essential adjunctive abilities for safe clinical practice.

Formal recognition of the roles and abilities of trainers has long been a feature of General Practice in the United Kingdom. The GMC is now introducing an analogous accreditation process for hospital practice, which will require recognised trainers to provide evidence that they deliver training to a defined standard.[5]

Curricula should never reach an endpoint of finalised stability. This would imply stagnation in development of clinical practice. The changes described above represent simply the latest in a continual change process that should reflect both the needs of clinical practice as it develops and the methods of delivering training as they improve. Complex interdependent relationships exist between service provision, curriculum writing, training and assessment methodology. It is clear, however, that collaboration between these components can result in effective improvement, which should contribute to improved patient care.

Key Point

- The 2013 surgical curriculum requires collation of documentary evidence of operative and important nonoperative skills. This forms a cornerstone for assessment of progression within training.

SELECTION INTO SURGICAL SPECIALTIES

Selection into all medical specialties in the United Kingdom underwent significant change with the launch of MMC and an associated computerised recruitment system known as the Medical Training Application Service (MTAS). Prior to this, all selection was carried out at a local or regional level with differing selection parameters and methodology. The traditional 20-minute interview with a panel of several interviewers asking unstructured questions was common. The process was inconsistent, inefficient due to many applicants applying for multiple advertised posts and open to accusations of favouritism and even nepotism.

MMC was revolutionary in its approach. Alongside the introduction of formal curricula for specialty training, a national selection process was initiated and attempts were made to introduce objective criteria into selection methodology. Unfortunately, not only was the selection design too generic and viewed as inappropriate for many specialties, but the computerised

MTAS system failed to cope with the volume of applications and the whole process collapsed. Nevertheless, many principles of the MMC selection process were valid and have subsequently been modified into a second-generation national selection methodology, which is now used by all surgical specialties in the United Kingdom.

The first task in designing a selection process for specialty training is to clarify the characteristics of the trainees required, who in turn will populate the consultant grade of the future. These characteristics should include a mixture of previous achievements, identifiable abilities and potential for future skill acquisition. With these in mind, a Person Specification is then drawn up listing essential criteria, that all applicants must meet, and desirable criteria, which are used to rank applicants.

The selection process is then designed to test all areas of the Person Specification. First, applicants who fail to meet the essential criteria on the application form are excluded, a process known colloquially as "long listing". Depending on the capacity of the selection process, it may then be possible to invite all applicants who meet the essential criteria to interview. However, if interview capacity is limited, then "short listing" is required. This uses the application form to examine desirable criteria and scores applicants to create a rank order from which the available interview slots are filled. The risk of short listing is that appointable applicants might be incorrectly excluded.

Given the challenges with short listing, all surgical specialties currently aim to carry out a face-to-face assessment of all applicants. Although this process is generally called the "interview", it is far removed from a traditional cross table assessment. "Selection Centre" is the proper term for the process, which includes a number of different assessments by different assessors, each testing a different aspect of the Person Specification. Each assessment is scored separately and it is recognised that the greater the number of individual assessments there are, the greater the reliability of the process. Each specialty has designed a slightly different process, but all aim to assess the breadth of the Person Specification.

A number of issues arise in the design of Selection Centres. A balance should be struck between assessing potential versus prior achievements. As selection processes do not have an upper limit of experience as an essential criterion (which would contravene the protected characteristic of age under equality legislation), trainees emerging from Core Surgical training are competing with others who have worked in the speciality for significantly longer. To adjust for this, a number of specialties include an upper limit of experience as a desirable criterion in their Person Specifications and then weight the scoring of previous achievements. These require more achievements from those who have been qualified longer.

All specialties currently include an assessment of technical skills. This increases the face validity of the process and has support from lay members. It is, however, the most difficult component to standardise and score reliably. A number of specialties include a communication element, using role-play with either an actor or assessor. This is often designed to place the applicant under a degree of stress to assess their ability to work under pressure (an essential criterion).

Some specialties use an applicant self-assessment system for scoring portfolios. This informs the assessment of experience, and the self-awarded scores are validated by the assessors. This has the advantage of transparency and to date has remained a useful tool despite the risk that trainees will, in time, work to meet all the top scoring criteria, so making this aspect of the assessment less useful. The issue of whether to publish the scoring criteria has been widely discussed. Some specialties publish full details, particularly of their methods of scoring portfolios of achievement. Others publish the domains, which are assessed in each component but not the descriptors for each score. It is difficult, however, to keep these descriptors privileged.

The question of assessor consistency, both for individual assessors (appropriately scoring applicants of differing abilities) and between assessors (assessing the same performance by an individual applicant) has been addressed in a number of ways. Assessment scenarios used are structured to provide material which can test differing levels of ability with each scenario accompanied by guidance notes for the assessors on how to conduct the conversation. The score sheets include different domains (mapped to the Person Specification) for every scenario with score descriptors for the type of performance expected for each score within the domains. This standardisation is further enhanced by assessor training, which in General Surgery, is carried out using an online training package.

The next stage of the development of national selection may be to examine the differences in the Person Specifications to identify whether it might be possible to align them more closely. In parallel to this, it may be possible to explore dividing selection into separate generic and specialty-specific components. This would have the theoretical advantage of further improving reliability of the process by increasing numbers and sharing ideas for the generic components whilst retaining individual specialty ownership through the specialty-specific sections. It may also be more cost-effective as the generic component could exclude the least competitive applicants who would then not be accommodated in the specialty-specific section.

What is clear from experience over the last seven years is that progress and improvements have been and are still being made by close involvement of enthusiastic trainers within each specialty. It is essential that future developments continue to have broad support and are not imposed.

Key Points

- Surgical training and assessment methodologies continually evolve. High-quality trainers and trainees should adapt to this.
- Selection Centre methodology utilises controlled exposure to multiple skill domains scored by a number of assessors to equitably rank specialty applicants at a national level.

SURGICAL TRAINING WITHIN MODERN WORKING REGULATIONS

In response to long working hours experienced by junior doctors in the United Kingdom in the 1980s, a "New Deal" was agreed between the British Medical Association and the Department of Health in 1991. This represented a contractual agreement for a 56-hour working week with a minimum of eight hours rest per day and a 30-minute break every four hours whilst at work. Punitive pay banding supplements were introduced in 2000 that incentivised National Health Service employers to bring working conditions into line with the New Deal, with full compliance required by August 2003.

The European Working Time Directive, adopted by the EU Council of Ministers in 1993[6] was intended to ensure safe working hours for individuals. It was introduced in the United Kingdom in 1998 and by August 2011, junior doctors were required to adhere to working 48 hours per week averaged over a six-month period. In addition, there was a requirement for one day of rest per week (or two per fortnight) and each working day had to include 11 hours of rest with a 20-minute break every six hours whilst at work. The SiMAP (Spain, 2000) and Jaeger (Germany, 2003) rulings from the European Court of Justice further defined that all time spent on site by an individual must be included for work and rest calculations, and secondly that this applied even if the individual was sleeping.

Today, consultants are subject to the ETWR but not the junior doctors' New Deal. Both the EWTR and New Deal must be adhered to by trainees in the United Kingdom, but they receive protection under whichever arrangements are more beneficial to them. As working hours are shorter under EWTR but rest breaks are more frequent under the New Deal, this results in a hybrid of the requirements to meet both regulations.

The Temple Report (2010) concluded that high-quality training can be delivered in 48 hours per week, but not where trainees have a major role in out-of-hours services, are poorly supervised and access to learning opportunities are limited.[7] The EWTRs have had a variable impact on doctors with an apparent disproportionate effect on surgical specialties. There is also continued debate as to whether patient safety has been improved as a result of full-shift EWTR compliant rotas, whether junior doctors' health and well-being has been affected and whether training has suffered. Some argue that problems exist because EWTR has not been implemented correctly, whereas others maintain that the system is so inflexible as to be incompatible with excellence and training.[8]

In April 2014, an independent working group, tasked by the Secretary of State for Health to assess the impact of the EWTR on patient safety and training, reported that EWTR had caused greater problems for certain specialties (surgery in particular) and that training in some acute specialties has been very difficult to deliver. Furthermore, local trusts have had mixed success in managing rotas to mitigate the effects of EWTR. Initial broad recommendations from the working group included reviewing best practice in training and sharing successful strategies between trusts, tackling the specific challenges faced by specialties most affected, addressing the lack of flexibility of EWTR, investigating the utility of individual opt-outs and assessing the feasibility of formally separating training and service provision by junior doctors.[9]

To mitigate against any potential deleterious effects of EWTR on training and continuity of patient care, and to respond to changing patient and disease demographics, it is now necessary to creatively tailor training and service commitments to ensure that trainees acquire appropriate skills and competencies to practice within a realistic professional framework at the point of substantive appointment.

Key Point

- To deliver high-quality training within EWTR, it is increasingly necessary to ensure training opportunities are maximised and appropriately balanced with service commitments to ensure that trainees acquire the necessary skills and competencies.

THE APPLICABILITY OF SURGICAL SIMULATION AND COURSES

Surgical simulation is both a valuable tool for safe acquisition of procedural skills in a nonclinical environment and also a potential strategy to mitigate the effects of the EWTR. Simulation is increasingly used in the selection of candidates into training programmes, as a component of their subsequent training, and also in assessment of progress. The ISCP General Surgery syllabus now includes simulation within PBAs and other specialties are now adopting a similar approach. As part of its 2013–2018 strategic aims, the Joint Committee on Surgical Training specifically aims to maximise the use of simulation techniques in surgical training and ensure that a robust system is in place for its quality assurance, justifying this as an essential step in improving patient safety.[10] Non-technical assessments within simulated clinical scenarios already form a key component of Intercollegiate examinations leading to Membership or Fellowship of one of the Royal Colleges of Surgeons (MRCS or FRCS respectively). There is a growing appetite for in-training assessment of competency as part of the Annual Review of Competence Progression (ARCP) process, but this has yet to be formalised due, in part, to the current heterogeneous provision of simulation facilities across the United Kingdom.

Simulation tools may be tailored to focus on operative or non-technical aspects of surgical practice. The clinical utility of simulation is well established. Multiple studies, meta-analyses and a recent Cochrane Review[11] of operative simulation studies have shown that simulation-based training (laparoscopic, endoscopic, and open surgery), as part of a structured programme and incorporating predetermined proficiency levels, results in skills transfer to the operative setting.[12]

In developing a surgical simulation curriculum, the validity of the simulator process should be known and the fidelity of simulators should be tailored to the desired educational outcomes. Commercially available products typically provide high-fidelity simulation but are expensive, and this inevitably impacts on accessibility. In essence, at an introductory level, where the primary goals focus on generic manual skills, fidelity appears less important. An example of this is low-resolution ureteroscopic simulator tools, which produce equivalent outcomes but are 185-times less expensive than high-fidelity commercial simulators.[13] Conversely, when practising specific operative procedures (such as laparoscopic colorectal surgery[14] and endovascular aneurysm repair[15]), high-fidelity tools are required. The most sophisticated simulator tools are able to replicate the exact anatomy of specific patients. Examples include endovascular aneurysm repair (EVAR) procedures or complex computer-assisted orthopaedic surgery using software that renders the computed tomography/magnetic resonance imaging into a simulator programme.

Within the United Kingdom, surgical simulation is currently predominantly delivered within the framework of dedicated training courses. These courses utilise procedural and nonoperative simulation tools to a variable extent. Many of the most successful simulation-based programmes aim to improve outcomes in nontechnical aspects of surgical practice. At one end of the spectrum lie programmes such as the Nontechnical Skills for Surgeons (NOTSS) and Care of the Critically Ill Surgical Patient (CCrISP) courses that focus on situational awareness, decision making and communication. Courses such as the Advanced Trauma Life Support (ATLS) course combine training and assessment of both nonprocedural and practical skills such as patient resuscitation and intravenous and airway access. Others make use of a graduated approach to realism—the basic upper gastrointestinal and basic colonoscopy courses, delivered by the Joint Advisory Group on Gastrointestinal Endoscopy provide lectures followed by low fidelity, then high fidelity simulators and culminating in supervised endoscopy on patients. A minority of courses have been identified as prerequisites for certification in specific procedures (e.g. accreditation to undertake independent endoscopy), and this is likely to increase as simulation becomes more widely available.

A radical approach to surgical training makes use of "boot camps" where trainees receive intensive simulation-based training prior to embarking upon clinical practice. This is most sophisticated in orthopaedic surgery, where early acquisition of technical skills is quicker in "boot camp" trainees compared to traditionally trained residents.[16] Furthermore, a modular competency-based curriculum (with frequent evaluations) in orthopaedic surgery appears to drive accelerated surgical competency, knowledge acquisition and professional skills.[17] These types of programmes are most definitely in the minority in surgical training across the world but appear promising (albeit expensive) avenues for accelerated training. Examples of adoption of "boot camp" type training courses in the United Kingdom include Cardiac Surgery programmes,[18] a Vascular Surgery boot camp for new appointees and the Highland General Surgical Boot Camp in Inverness, Scotland.[19]

Surgical simulation, within short courses, longer boot camps or as part of a modular and regularly assessed curriculum, should be encouraged to provide safe operative and nontechnical skills acquisition for surgical trainees. For surgical simulation to become widely available in both formative and summative assessment formats, a co-ordinated national scheme is likely to be required to ensure equity of access, consistency of quality, validity of methodology and also value for money.

Key Points

- Surgical simulation enables the safe acquisition of operative and non-technical skills. The fidelity of simulation should be tailored to the specific goals of trainees at different stages of training. Increased availability of simulation tools should permit broader incorporation of simulation into UK training programmes.
- Future surgical curricula may make use of dedicated periods spent within formal simulation environments ("boot camps") as a novel, accelerated training programme methodology.

REFERENCES

1. Smith MK. (1996, 2000). 'Curriculum theory and practice' the encyclopaedia of informal education. [online] Available from www.infed.org/biblio/b-curric.htm.
2. The Intercollegiate Surgical Curriculum 2013—General Surgery. [online] Available from http://www.gmc-uk.org/General_Surgery__Simulation_Curriculum__Aug_20131.pdf_56003282.pdf

3. Securing the future of excellent patient care. Final report of the independent review led by Professor David Greenaway. SOT/SFEPC/1013. October 2013. [online] Available from http://www.shapeoftraining.co.uk/static/documents/content/Shape_of_training_FINAL_Report.pdf_53977887.pdf.

4. Workplace based assessments. Intercollegiate surgical curriculum programme. [online] Available from https://www.iscp.ac.uk/surgical/assessment_wba.aspx.

5. Recognising and approving trainers: the implementation plan. General Medical Council. August 2012. [online] Available from http://www.gmc-uk.org/Approving_trainers_implementation_plan_Aug_12.pdf_56452109.pdf.

6. Directive 2003/88/EC of the European Parliament and of the Council of 4 November 2003 concerning certain aspects of the organisation of working time. Official Journal L 299. 2003;0009-19.

7. Temple J. Time for training: a review of the impact of the EWTD on the quality of training. 2010. http://hee.nhs.uk/healtheducationengland/files/2012/08/Time-for-training-report.pdf.

8. Williams N. EWTD revisited. Ann R Coll Surg Engl (Suppl). 2014;96:140-1.

9. Independent Working Time Regulations Taskforce Report to the Department of Health. The implementation of the Working Time Directive and its impact on the NHS and health professionals. 2014. http://www.rcseng.ac.uk/policy/documents/wtd-taskforce-report-2014.

10. The Joint Committee on Specialist Training: JCST Strategy 2013-18. [online] Available from http://www.jcst.org/key-documents/docs/jcst-strategy-2013-18.

11. Gurusamy KS, Aggarwal R, Palanivelu L, et al. Virtual reality training for surgical trainees in laparoscopic surgery. Cochrane Database Syst Rev. 2009(1):CD006575.

12. Dawe SR, Pena GN, Windsor JA, et al. Systematic review of skills transfer after simulation-based training. Brit J Surg. 2014;101(9):1063-76.

13. Brunckhorst O, Aydin A, Aboudi H, et al. Simulation-based ureteroscopy training: a systematic review. J Surg Educ. 2014. doi:10.1016/j.surg.2014.07.003. Epub ahead of print.

14. Miskovic D, Wyles SM, Ni M, et al. Systematic review on mentoring and simulation in laparoscopic colorectal surgery. Ann Surg. 2010;252(6):943-51.

15. Davis GR, Illig KA, Yang G, et al. An approach to EVAR simulation using patient specific modelling. Ann Vasc Surg. 2014. doi: 10.1016/j.avsg.2014.05.007 (Epub ahead of print).

16. Sonnadara RR, van Vliet A, Safir O, et al. Orthopedic boot camp: Examining the effectiveness of an intensive surgical skills course. Surgery. 2011;149(6):745-9.

17. Ferguson PC, Kraemer W, Nousiainen M, et al. Three-year experience with an innovative, modular, competency-based curriculum for orthopaedic training. J Bone Joint Surg Am. 2013; 6;95(21):e166. doi: 10.2106/JBJS.M.00314.

18. Macfie RC, Webel AD, Nesbitt JC, et al. "Boot camp" simulator training in open hilar dissection in early cardiothoracic surgical residency. Ann Thoracic Surg. 2014;97(1):161-6.

19. Hamlin K, Finlayson D. Highland surgical boot camp—an apprenticeship in a week. BMJ Careers 14 April 2012. http://careers.bmj.com/careers/advice/view-article.html?id=20007091.

2

Chapter

Confidential Reporting Systems in Surgical Practice

Frank CT Smith, Adam M Lewis, Denis C Wilkins

INTRODUCTION

"To err is human. To cover up is unforgivable. To fail to learn is inexcusable".

Liam Donaldson, Chief Medical Officer, 2004

In recent years there has been increasing concern about patient safety in the United Kingdom and worldwide. Despite best efforts, the incidence of adverse events, surgical mishaps and "near misses" in UK hospitals remains significant.

In 2007, for instance, 129,416 surgical errors were reported to the national patient safety agency (NPSA) and 1,136 operative errors occurred. In a study reported from Aberdeen during the same period, it was estimated that one in seven patients suffered an adverse event whilst in hospital. In 2011/12 the national health service (NHS) Litigation Authority reported payouts of £729.1 million for clinical negligence claims, a surrogate marker underestimating the volume of adverse events incurred by NHS patients, and in 2013/14 there were 261 reported surgical "Never Events", including 123 instances of retained foreign objects at surgery; 49 wrong implants or prostheses and 89 incidents of wrong-side surgery.

Whilst it is recognised that adverse events and surgical mishaps will never be completely eradicated from clinical practice, it is vital that effective systems for reporting adverse events exist to educate and inform surgeons and surgical teams of potential pitfalls, aiming to help them avoid these problems, with concomitant benefits for patient safety.

This chapter describes the principal confidential reporting systems for surgery in the United Kingdom and outlines their relative merits and limitations.

CONFIDENTIAL REPORTING: LESSONS FROM AVIATION

Confidential reporting implies that an individual brings to the attention of a body, completely independent of the management influences, information relevant to safety, but with the reassurance that the reporter's identity remains confidential to that body alone. The information may relate to adverse incidents, "near misses", inadequacies of the reporter, peers, or the organisation that they represent, or a regulatory authority.

In aviation, reporting of certain adverse circumstances to the appropriate regulatory authorities is mandatory, but voluntary systems allowing employees to inform their individual companies of potential problems also exist. The latter may have limitations in providing information with respect to management inadequacies and behavioural traits, and this led to the introduction of confidential reporting in the aviation industry.[1]

Confidentiality, NOT anonymity, and independence from the external pressures of management, form the essentials of such a reporting system. It was this premise that led to the formation of the UK confidential air human factors incident reporting programme (CHIRP). The instigators of this programme have commented on the initial resistance to the concept by airline management and regulatory authorities, concerned that such a system might flag up alleged deficiencies in their own procedures. Nonetheless, since CHIRP came into being in 1982, in the intervening 32 years, the organisation has come to be accepted as a mainstay for provision of safety information for general aviation in the United Kingdom.

When the Association of Surgeons of Great Britain and Ireland (ASGBI) first muted the question of setting up an analogous confidential reporting system for surgery (CORESS), advice was obtained from the chief executive and Board of CHIRP. At the inception of the CORESS, the Chief Executive of CHIRP was invited to sit on the CORESS Board and liaison between the organisations has since provided a valuable source of procedural support to the surgical reporting system.

Key Points

- Errors need to be recorded and analysed if we are to discover how they could have been prevented.
- People will report error if conditions are right.

THE CONFIDENTIAL REPORTING SYSTEM FOR SURGERY

The Confidential Reporting System for Surgery[2,3] was initially set up under the auspices of the ASGBI in 2006, but in 2010 it became an independent charity, introduced by Sir Bruce Keogh, NHS Medical Director at its launch at the House of Lords. It differs from other reporting systems in that it was specifically set up by surgeons for the benefit of surgeons, (and patients), and the surgical fraternity.

The mission statement of CORESS is "to feedback widely to the surgical community and elsewhere, the learning contained in reports of surgical accidents, errors, mishaps and "near miss" events, in a manner which is effective but which preserves the confidentiality of the reporter and his or her institution of origin".

Although there are differences between aviation and surgery, the principles underlying confidential reporting systems are the same.[4] Firstly, there must be complete confidentiality between reporter and system to encourage submission of reports and to attenuate perceptions of existence of a blame culture. Confidentiality is not the same as anonymity. The reporter's identity must be known to the organisation so that verification and, if necessary, elaboration of incident details may be undertaken. However, knowledge of the contributor's details should be kept to a minimum subset, and in the case of CORESS, these details are known to the programme director alone.

Secondly, published reports must have an educational value, with credible feedback to the reporter and to the profession. The feedback from CORESS is produced by a pan-specialty Advisory Board with representatives from all of the surgical specialty associations, who are practicing surgeons. Other members of the Advisory Board comprise lay people, surgical trainees, nurses, legal representatives, members with human factors expertise, representatives of the Royal Colleges, and of the medical defence organisations. The Board is independent of any authority and is led by the programme director who acts as an independent chair and is not remunerated by the organisation. An important point is that advisors are appointed to the Advisory Board to provide expert opinion and NOT to represent the interests of their organisations.

Lastly, confidence in the system by those interested but not directly involved is necessary. The reporting system is complementary to existing mandatory reporting systems, and to existing statutory, professional and organisational measures for the protection of the public. It does not replace them.

Any surgeon, surgical trainee or member of the operating department may submit a case to CORESS, either by hard copy, or via an on-line reporting form which can be downloaded at www.coress.org.uk. Previously, published reports can also be downloaded from the website and a database enabling search and retrieval of cases using search key words is under construction. In a move to encourage reporting rates, reporters are provided with a Certificate of Contribution, which can be included in the reporter's continuing professional development portfolio for appraisal, revalidation or training purposes.

Reports may concern any safety-related incident involving the reporter, other people, hospitals or clinical organisations that the reporter deals with. Incidents may include diagnostic or surgical errors, technical or maintenance failures, regulatory or procedural aspects, unsafe practices and protocols. Recent reports have related to medications, devices, injection errors,

Flowchart 2.1: Confidential reporting system for surgery report management process.

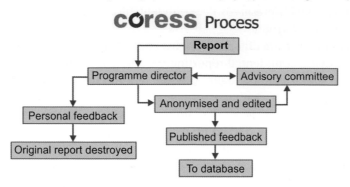

and to communication and hand-over failures. Useful lessons may be learnt from "near misses", and incidents, which have not resulted in adverse consequences, the details of which may be known only to the reporter. However, there is no educational value in reporting incidents from which no lesson can be learned.[3] Incidents with no safety content or relating to personality conflicts, to human resource issues, or to terms and conditions of employment or industrial relations are not generally useful.

Flowchart 2.1 illustrates how confidential reports received by CORESS are dealt with. Confidentiality is the fundamental concept underpinning the CORESS service. On receipt of a report it is transferred to a stand-alone computer with no network, wireless or Internet connections. The programme director, who removes all identifying details, which may connect the report to a specific patient, department or institution, reviews the report. It is then passed to the expert Advisory Board, members of which have all signed a confidentiality agreement. If the Board agrees that lessons can be learned, these are teased out and an unidentifiable version is included in a feedback report for publication.

Publication of CORESS reports is undertaken routinely in the Annals of the Royal College of Surgeons of England, Surgeons' News, the Journal of the Royal College of Surgeons of Edinburgh, and the Journal of the Association of Surgeons of Great Britain and Ireland. The Royal College of Ophthalmologists has recently adopted the reporting system and publishes ophthalmology reports in their journal. Specialty-specific reports have also been published for instance, in Vascular Society and ENT newsletters, and in the Journal of Hand Surgery. Smaller condensed reports, "CORESS-Lite" bytes, have also been circulated electronically.

The reporter is provided with the Advisory Board's comments as feedback, and with information confirming the proposed outcome. All identifying data are deleted from the system before publication of a report.

In a spirit of cooperation to advance surgical safety, whilst maintaining strict confidentiality, CORESS is represented on the Surgical Patient Safety

Expert Group of NHS England, and contributed to the publication of the NHS England "Never Events" Task Force Report[5] published in February 2014.

CORESS contributes to surgical safety by publication of relevant educational vignettes for practicing surgeons. Each vignette tells a story and has undergone root cause analysis. The organisation does not attempt to replicate mandatory reporting mechanisms or large systematic analyses on the scale of incident reporting by NHS organisations such as the National Reporting and Learning Service (NRLS). There is no point in replicating these necessary projects. Rather, CORESS complements these official systems, providing relevant feedback to individual surgeons and to the surgical community at large.

The epithet: "There, but for the grace of God, go I", is a powerful educational tool for the surgeon, particularly in an era when public scrutiny is increasingly (and rightly) intolerant of surgical mistakes and adverse outcomes. In an appropriate aviation analogy, the Royal Observer Corps' motto "Forewarned is forearmed" might equally apply to lessons learned from voluntary confidential reporting in surgery.

NATIONAL CONFIDENTIAL ENQUIRY INTO PATIENT OUTCOMES AND DEATHS (NCEPOD)

The NCEPOD[6] was set up following a confidential and anonymous pilot study of mortality associated with anaesthesia, undertaken by Lunn and Mushin[7] in 1982. The organisation, with the initial appellation, CEPOD, was a joint venture between anaesthetic and surgical specialties, which reviewed surgical and anaesthetic practice over one year in three health-care regions. In 1988, NCEPOD was established with Government funding and with an initial interest focused solely on surgical outcomes, in which the organisational nomenclature referred to the National Confidential Enquiry into Perioperative Deaths. Its first report was published in 1990. Since its inception however, in recent years, the organisation's title has morphed again, into that reflected at the heading of this section. NCEPOD now covers all specialties, as a direct result of its need to secure continued funding, and the surgical focus of the organisation and the relevance of all studies to surgeons, has been diluted somewhat.

The NCEPOD's purpose is to assist in improving standards of medical and surgical care, by reviewing the management of patients in specific clinical spheres, through commissioned confidential surveys and research. A published report is generated for each topic review.

The NCEPOD analyses aspects of current practice within a specialty field in which, typically, there are not always agreed standards. Recent reports of interest to surgeons have included aortic aneurysm surgery, bariatric surgery and in 2014, amputations. Data are acquired according to carefully constructed questionnaires relating to individual patients, to provide a prolonged "snapshot" of patient management over a given period. The studies do not seek to analyse new treatments, to undertake prospective research, or to allocate patients to treatment groups. Each year NCEPOD invites study proposals for forthcoming work. These proposals have to be relevant to the current clinical environment and to have potential to inform debate with respect to service improvement for patient benefit. Studies are commissioned by the healthcare quality improvement programme (HQIP).

The NCEPOD publishes its studies as full reports and as summaries. These are sent to Local Reporters for onwards dissemination to consultants and other health-care professionals within their hospitals. NCEPOD is independent of government bodies and professional associations. It is both a charity and a company limited by guarantee. The organisation has a key role to make recommendations for care at local clinical level, but also with respect to service provision at local and national levels. A Board of Directors governs NCEPOD, but the body's work and standards are overseen by a Steering Group. Members include nominated representatives of the Royal Colleges and Associations, as well as lay and nursing representation. Observers representing HQIP, and the Coroner's Society attend meetings, ensuring clinical integrity of the work undertaken. Reports tend to provide recommendations with respect to organisational care, and recent surgical reports have included recommendations with respect to preoperative, peri-, and postoperative care. A long-standing recommendation exists for the use of audit as a means of identifying remediable factors in patient care at local level.

A multidisciplinary group of experts is responsible for contributing to the design of each study and for reviewing findings and producing recommendations. The process concentrates on aspects of remediable care for patients in the clinical area under consideration. The study population is clearly defined and organisational data are obtained from participating hospitals. Within each hospital a named contact, the NCEPOD Local Reporter, is identified, providing a link between NCEPOD and hospital staff, facilitating case identification, dissemination of questionnaires and data collection. Data for the study population are collected via comprehensive questionnaires, which are completed by the clinicians responsible for the care of those patients. The study patient population is identified by OPCS and ICD10 codes. Case note extraction is undertaken and a multidisciplinary group of advisors undertakes peer review of a sample of case notes and associated questionnaires, for quality control purposes. All patient identifiers are removed prior to review. Qualitative and quantitative data summaries are derived and reviewed by expert authors and the Steering Group to inform the final recommendations of a report.

Since its inception, NCEPOD recommendations have been instrumental in significant changes in organisational behaviour and service provision, improving patient safety and the delivery of care in the United Kingdom.

Key Point

- For surgeons and clinical staff to have faith in a reporting system, transparent, robust and rigorously enforced mechanisms must exist to ensure confidentiality of reports.

THE NPSA AND THE NRLS

The NPSA was a special health authority of the NHS in England, established in 2001, to monitor patient safety incidents, including medication and prescribing errors in the NHS. Its remit grew over time to include, in 2005, overseeing safety aspects of hospital design, and safety in medical research, through the Central Office for Research Ethics. Between 2005 and 2012, it hosted the National Clinical Assessment Service, which aimed to resolve concerns about the performance of individual doctors and dentists. Finally, it also managed contracts with the three confidential enquiry services, [NCEPOD, Confidential Enquiry into Maternal and Child Health (CEMACH); Confidential Enquiry into Suicide and Homicide (CISH)], before devolving this responsibility to the National Institute for Health and Clinical Excellence.

The NPSA was established to ensure that incidents were reported, but also to promote an open and fair culture in hospitals and across the health services, encouraging doctors and other staff to report incidents and "near misses". The aim was to develop a no-blame culture and to encourage staff to report without fear of personal reprimand or reprisal, enabling others to learn from those experiences for the benefit of patient safety.

The NPSA developed the NRLS,[8] to collect and analyse information from patients and staff. From 2005 onwards, it has been possible for NHS staff to submit safety incident information through web-based forms (Fig. 2.1), although roll out of the system took 2 years longer than originally envisaged. The reporting form can be found at http://www.nrls.npsa.nhs.uk.

The NRLS receives confidential reports of patient safety incidents from health-care staff across England and Wales. These reports are analysed by clinicians and safety experts to identify common risks to patients and opportunities to improve patient safety. NRLS outputs include Patient Safety Alerts, (including Rapid Response reports cascaded to NHS staff); the "Seven Steps" series of patient safety guides; feedback on data collected and safety information on specific topics. It has been suggested that organisations with a higher rate of reporting incidents have a stronger safety culture. Information from safety incidents is used to develop guidance tools and campaigns to encourage NHS organisations to learn from incidents, reducing risk of future recurrence.

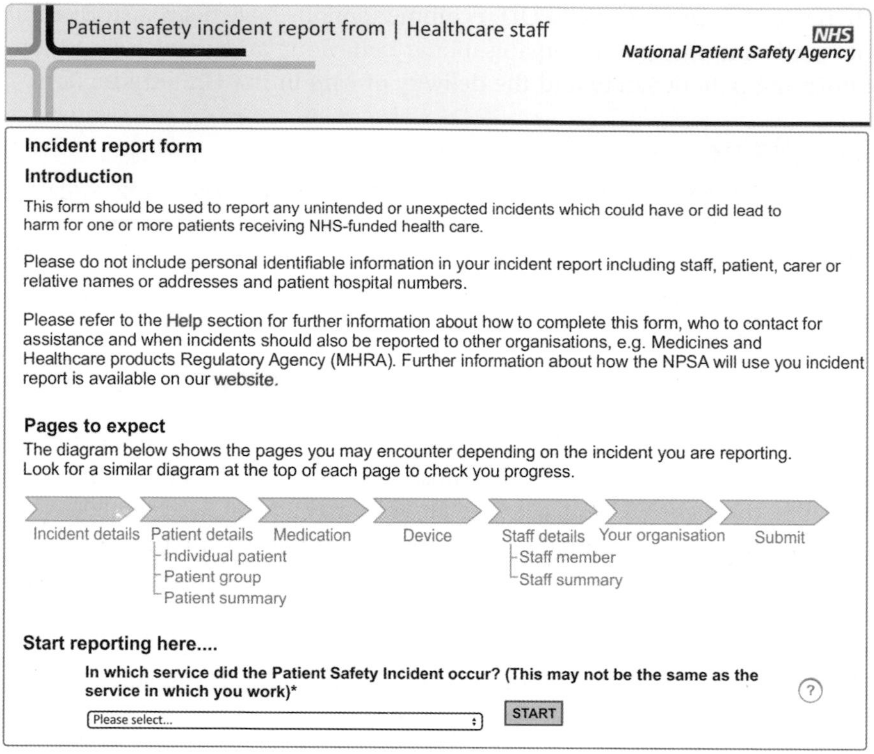
Patient safety incident report from | Healthcare staff

NHS
National Patient Safety Agency

Incident report form

Introduction

This form should be used to report any unintended or unexpected incidents which could have or did lead to harm for one or more patients receiving NHS-funded health care.

Please do not include personal identifiable information in your incident report including staff, patient, carer or relative names or addresses and patient hospital numbers.

Please refer to the Help section for further information about how to complete this form, who to contact for assistance and when incidents should also be reported to other organisations, e.g. Medicines and Healthcare products Regulatory Agency (MHRA). Further information about how the NPSA will use you incident report is available on our website.

Pages to expect

The diagram below shows the pages you may encounter depending on the incident you are reporting. Look for a similar diagram at the top of each page to check you progress.

Incident details
Patient details
- Individual patient
- Patient group
- Patient summary
Medication
Device
Staff details
- Staff member
- Staff summary
Your organisation
Submit

Start reporting here....

In which service did the Patient Safety Incident occur? (This may not be the same as the service in which you work)*

Please select...
START

Fig. 2.1: National reporting and learning service electronic incident report form (http://www.nrls.npsa.nhs.uk)

A problem for individual clinicians has been in isolating relevant information from the large volume of cases assimilated by the NRLS, most of which are not relevant to an individual surgeon's practice. For instance, 612,414 safety incidents were reported to the NRLS between October 2011 and March 2012. Contributions were received from 90% of NHS Trusts in England. Of these, in 68%, no harm came to the patient; in 25% low harm was incurred; in 6% there was moderate harm; 1% of incidents resulted in death or severe harm. The most common types of incident reported were: patient accidents, slips, trips and falls (26%); medication incidents (11%); incidents related to treatments or procedures (11%). These figures were consistent with previous data releases.

Despite good intentions, there were significant criticisms of the NPSA. In 2006, the Government White Paper, "Safety First",[9] commissioned by the Chief Medical Officer, Sir Liam Donaldson, noted "a high volume of incidents reports..." but, "...too few examples where these had resulted in actionable learning for NHS organisations". Furthermore, it was recognised that there was "...little evidence that data collected through the National

Reporting and Learning Service are effectively informing patient safety at local NHS level".

In 2009, the House of Commons Health Committee on Patient Safety[10] made further critical comments: "Despite great strides made in incident reporting, its effectiveness is limited by significant under-reporting; absence of a fair blame culture in the NHS; lack of focus in the NRLS..." *and suggested that there were* "... inherent limitations of data from reporting systems as a means of generating information about patient safety issues and solutions".

The jury, therefore, is still out on the value of large scale incident reporting and the inherent difficulties in extracting relevant and meaningful data remain unresolved. In 2012, the NPSA was abolished and its key functions including the NRLS were transferred to the NHS Commissioning Board Special Heath Authority.

Key Points

- Educational benefits of confidential reporting are best achieved in a blame-free culture.
- Effective feedback is an essential component of confidential reporting.

CONCLUSION

In 2005, the Scottish Audit of Surgical Mortality[11] summarised the need for medical participation in confidential incident reporting with the following statements:

"There is agreement that our healthcare system needs to transform the existing culture of blame and punishment that suppresses information about errors into a positive culture focused on patient safety and quality improvement. The lessons learned in aviation support this view.[12]

Clinicians are encouraged to report and evaluate medical error, if they are within a safe learning environment. When clinicians can report error in a voluntary and confidential manner, everyone benefits.

Voluntary data gathering systems are more effective than mandatory systems in promoting improvement as a result of the lessons learnt from audit".

This chapter has outlined current aspects of confidential reporting of patient safety incidents and has described reporting systems in the United Kingdom. Other reporting systems, specific to institutions, exist within individual NHS hospitals. Such systems and the lessons learned from each are complementary. Taken together, the educational elements derived from confidential reporting should serve to influence and improve surgical, organisational and systems-related aspects of surgical care, with resultant benefits for patient safety in our health-care systems.

Key Points

- Useful lessons may be learnt from "near misses", and incidents, which have not resulted in adverse consequences.
- Voluntary confidential reporting systems are complementary to, and do NOT replace mandatory reporting systems.

REFERENCES

1. Nicholson AN, Tait PC. Confidential reporting: from aviation to clinical medicine. Clin Med JRCPL. 2002;2:234-6.
2. http://www.coress.org.uk. 2014.
3. Lewis AM, Taylor I. CORESS—a confidential reporting system for surgery. Ann R Coll Surg Engl. 2006;88(3):249-51.
4. Lewis AM, Smith FCT, Tait P, et al. UK surgery already applies aviation safety practice. BMJ. 2011;342:d1310.
5. Standardise Educate, Harmonise. Commissioning the Conditions for Safer Surgery. Report of the NHS England Never Events Task Force. Feb 2014. Available from http://www.england.nhs.uk/wp-content/uploads/2014/02/sur-nev-ev-tf-rep.pdf. 2014.
6. http://www.ncepod.org.uk. 2014.
7. Lunn JN, Mushin WW. Mortality associated with anaesthesia. Anaesthesia. 1982;37(8):856.
8. http://www.nrls.npsa.nhs.uk. 2014.
9. Department of Health. Safety first: a report for patients, clinicians and healthcare managers. 2006. Available from http://webarchive.nationalarchives.gov.uk. 2014.
10. House of Commons Health Committee. Patient Safety. Sixth Report of Session 2008–09. London: The Stationery Office Limited; 2009, vol I. HC 151-I.
11. Qualified Confidentiality, Patient safety and Freedom of Information. Discussion Paper, Scottish Audit of Surgical Mortality 2005. http://www.sasm.org.uk. 2014.
12. Berwick D, Leape L. Reducing errors in medicine. It's time to take this more seriously. BMJ. 1999;319:136-47.

3

Chapter

The Management of Knife Injuries

Miss C Webster, Lt Col Nigel Tai

PHILOSOPHY OF APPROACH

Death from trauma accounts for 30% of all life years lost in the United States,[1] and is the third leading cause of death in 15–29 year olds in Europe.[2] Penetrating trauma (Fig. 3.1) appears to be increasing in the United Kingdom, with an annual increase of patients sustaining stab wounds at 23.2% at one major London National Health Service (NHS) trust[3] therefore remaining a significant public health issue.

The architecture of care for trauma patients in England has undergone dramatic change, due to the creation of designated trauma networks, with NHS England Commissioners accountable for their processes and outcomes of care. Standards are set by a national, multi-disciplinary board (the Clinical Reference Group for Trauma) and monitored through peer review visits, process-of-care dashboards and predictive mortality modelling based upon compulsorily collected patient data.

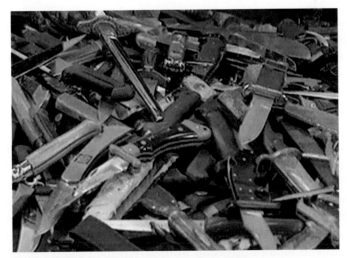

Fig. 3.1: Confiscated knives in the Scottish Courts in 2009.
Source: http://news.stv.tv/scotland/222108-more-than-2000-knives-were-seized-in-scottish-courts-last-year/.

Management of a patient with a stab wound should begin at the point of injury, with appropriate road-side triage and either rapid transport to the nearest major trauma centre or mobilisation of an enhanced pre-hospital response centred on physician-delivered pre-hospital emergency care (PHEC).[4] Most stab wounds require no emergent intervention, but recognition of the sick patient who presents with evidence of tension pneumothorax, cardiac tamponade or catastrophic haemorrhage (from extremity, torso or junctional area) provides an opportunity to either treat at the scene or rapidly transport the patient. Pre-hospital emergency care-trained physicians can choose the correct path for their patient, with deployment of advanced airway skills (which have been deemed an essential skill for pre-hospital doctors),[5] circulatory access and the application of haemostatic dressings and tourniquets in order to sustain the patients physiology as required. Pre-hospital resuscitative thoracotomy is established in many regions as a technique that can be effective in restoring circulatory output in the management of cardiac tamponade, though survival rates for thoracotomy in exsanguination (using an aortic cross clamp) are dismal.[6] Based on the experience of UK Defence Medical Services, some PHEC systems have made en route pre-hospital transfusion of blood and plasma available to PHEC providers, although the evidence that this affects outcome has yet to be conclusively demonstrated.[7] Pre-hospital use of tranexamic acid is increasingly part of the management of the bleeding, stabbed patient.[8,9] These elements of trauma management are termed damage control resuscitation (DCR).[10] It begins at the roadside, encompasses surgical management and critical care, and is aimed at preserving and restoring physiology first and foremost.

Unless the patient is in absolute extremis, the British Trauma Networks are predicated upon bypass of local smaller hospitals in favour of transport to the more replete setting of the designated Major Trauma Centre. The evidence supporting this strategy is well established.[11,12] Major Trauma Centres are commissioned centrally to provide standards of trauma care that are appropriate for the management of severely injured patients—this should include 24/7 consultant presence in the emergency department (ED), and a multi-disciplinary trauma team with all relevant expertise (including access to vascular and cardiothoracic specialists). Rapid access to on-site whole body computed tomography (CT), expedited transfusion services, interventional radiology and emergency theatre are other mandatory features. Reception and evaluation of the major trauma patient must occur hand-in-hand with ongoing volume resuscitation, with abbreviation of normal ED processes and prompt diversion to theatre if the patient's instability merits emergent laparotomy, thoracotomy or vascular control. Clear standard operation procedures and appropriate team simulation can be valuable in fostering the right behaviours and team manoeuvres.

Key Point

- Surgeons practicing in major trauma centres and trauma units must understand, and contribute to, the local operating procedures governing the function of their local trauma system. Familiarity with reception, triage and onwards movement protocols will ensure that they can deliver their assigned role to best effect.

IMMEDIATE ASSESSMENT AND INVESTIGATION

The patient should be assessed by the Trauma Team (Fig. 3.2) in standard CABC fashion, where identification and treatment of immediate threats to life are carried out concurrently. (C)atastrophic haemorrhage is identified and dealt with primarily (e.g. application of a tourniquet, direct pressure or decision to proceed to emergent intervention for non-compressible haemorrhage), followed by assessment and management of (A)irway, (B)reathing and (C)irculation. Stab wounds can be the result of an assault, self-infliction—or rarely an accident—the circumstances of the injury should be elucidated but are usually not relevant to the immediate resuscitation. Wounds may be isolated, few or many, but all must be systematically identified, mapped and assessed for likelihood of breach of underlying cavities or structures. Probing a wound with your digits or a surrogate is painful for an awake patient and, if a cavity cannot be directly sounded, a "negative" result may simply reflect the muscles of the torso acting to "baffle" the wound track. The back, axillae, buttock folds, groins and infra-mammary areas should not be overlooked. Do not be deceived by a small entry wound, as this describes nothing about the depth of the wound. Similarly, information regarding the weapon is useful—sometimes it will be brought

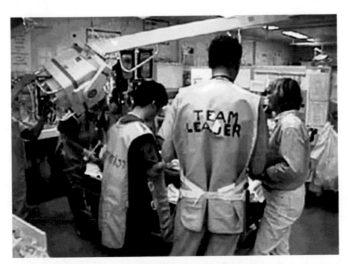

Fig. 3.2: A Typical Trauma Team in the Emergency Department.
Source: www.trauma.org.

with the patient—but do not feel reassured by a short weapon as even these knives can penetrate deeply with sufficient force. Remember any weapon is evidenced and must be handed to the police with minimal handling. The patient will often arrive with a police escort. They will ask about the clinical details of the patient for purposes of charging a potential suspect. This confidential information can be given to the police, but can be basic, e.g. "life threatening" or "life changing" injuries. Remember this to be a patient with an injury and under no circumstances whatsoever should judgment be exercised. The patient will be frightened; reassure them.

It is a truism that the young are able to preserve their blood pressure until catastrophic collapse is eventually encountered but one that must be continually mitigated through constant consideration of compensation when assessing the stab victim. This is especially the case if effective PHEC has masked the underlying seriousness of the physiological disturbance. Whilst haemorrhage is implicated in approximately 30% of pre-hospital deaths[13] advanced pre-hospital resuscitation has been shown to improve outcomes.[14] Some of the newer techniques have emigrated from recent experience of Defence Medical Services in Afghanistan although the utility of these measures has yet to be well evidenced for UK civil society:

- Bilateral/Unilateral Thoracostomy. This manoeuvre is practiced in the pre-hospital domain by PHEC physician responders when there is clinical suspicion of tension pneumothorax as part of the "Rule Out" approach to the unstable trauma patient. About 1–2 cm incisions are made in the "safe triangle" bilaterally which are the port for the later insertion of the chest drain.

- Tourniquets (Fig. 3.3). Whilst direct firm pressure is usually enough to staunch limb bleeding, the application of a tourniquet is more practical and allows for patient transport. The Combat Application Tourniquet is increasingly popular, and has certainly influenced survival in the battle casualty, however, civilian data also supports their use in penetrating vascular injury.[15] Minor morbidity from the use of a tourniquet is acknowledged (e.g. limb shortening, nerve palsy at the application site, pain and kidney injury); however, the benefit in improved survival rates in major haemorrhage mean that's use is still advocated in appropriate circumstances.[16] If a patient arrives with a tourniquet in situ, note the application time, check whether it is applied tightly (it should be) and whether bleeding is controlled. If the wound is still bleeding, tighten the tourniquet by the minimal amount required to gain haemostasis. Be aware that a wound beneath a loosely applied tourniquet may not bleed until the circulating volume has been restored. If the wound is judged to not involve a vascular structure, a tourniquet can be loosened, but only under direct observation of the wound to ensure that it declares itself and the tourniquet retightened if your judgment is incorrect. Tourniquets should be removed as soon as possible once you are in a position to confirm that either the wound does not pose a threat

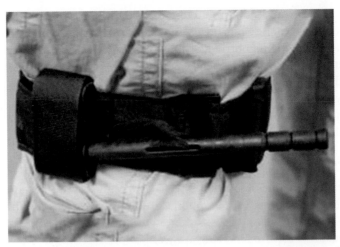

Fig. 3.3: The Combat Applicator Tourniquet (CAT) used in significant military and civilian limb haemorrhage.
Source: www.aidtraining.co.uk.

of catastrophic haemorrhage or vascular control has been obtained. It is rare for a pre-hospital tourniquet time to be longer than an hour in the United Kingdom.

- Novel haemostatic agents. Some Ambulance Services and PHEC physicians have access to haemostatic dressing such as Celox for use on relatively superficial wounds although these are not licensed for use in chest, abdominal or cranial cavities.[17] Wounds packed with such dressing should be explored in the anaesthetized patient in an operating theatre and not disturbed until that point less unwise probing lead to the de-roofing of a contained haemorrhage.

- Open thoracotomy (clamshell) wound. PHEC physicians are increasingly trained in this manoeuvre as a result of essential cadaveric courses.[18] The chest will have been opened for one of three pathologies—pericardial tamponade or exsanguinating thoracic or abdominal trauma.[19,20] If it is the former and the patient has a circulatory output, it is because the PHEC doctor has drained the pericardium and applied a haemostatic myocardial suture. The correct surgical response is to take the patient to theatre, to evaluate the heart, mediastinal and thoracic contents for other injuries and treat as required, and to close the thoracotomy wound in an appropriate manner. For patients with high grade blood loss secondary to exsanguination from any site, an aortic clamp or aortic manual pressure may have been applied in order to preserve flow to the myocardium and brain. There will have been little opportunity for the PHEC doctor to do more than this and rule out a tamponade. The burden of intervention will fall to the surgeon, and the correct response is to initiate massive volume transfusion via a central line (or the right atrium) and take the patient directly to theatre for control of bleeding from the pulmonary structures or intra-abdominal viscera as directed by surgical interrogation of the breached compartment. In either case—drained tamponade or uncontrolled haemorrhage—the arrival of a pre-hospital thoracotomy patient who is in asystole suggests that further effort is futile.[21]

In MTCs the use of "Code Red" Resuscitation protocols for massively bleeding patients has become established as a means of co-ordinating trauma team and surgical responses. Flowchart 3.1 gives the Royal London Hospital Code Red protocol.

Key Point

- The ED reception of the stabbed patient should focus on CABC and should be organised along defined trauma team roles. An increasing armoury of pre-hospital treatment can be used, many of which have implications for the receiving surgeon.

INVESTIGATION

Triaging the body cavities for haemorrhage is the sequence of diagnostic manoeuvres used to locate the compelling source of bleeding. A deteriorating, unstable patient with penetrating torso trauma is best investigated in the operating theatre with the treating surgeon basing his or her operative strategy on the outcome of initial chest X-ray and focused assessment by sonography for trauma scan; however, there is certainly a merited place for CT scanning of certain groups of patients. Computed tomography can provide valuable information on whether mediastinal injuries have been sustained, on whether a vascular injury has occurred, and whether the abdominal cavity has been violated.[22] Where the configuration of knife wound track and underlying solid organ injury is confirmed—with no evidence of any intervening hollow viscus—a conservative management strategy may be selected if there is no contrast blush or pseudo-aneurysm appearance. Presence of these latter features can guide the surgeon to seek angio-embolisation.

RESUSCITATION

Damage control resuscitation aims to correct the well-described lethal triad of trauma (hypothermia, acidosis and coagulopathy) with appropriate transfusion of packed cells and blood plasma, patient warming, optimal oxygenation and damage control surgery. Without this, mortality of the named "Lethal Triad" (Fig. 3.4) is almost 50%.[23] It is a concept that has been reinforced by military experience in Iraq and Afghanistan, but there is a growing consensus of opinion and civilian evidence that this approach translates to improved survival.[24] The use of Belmont and Level One type infusers allows rapid restoration of circulating volume. Crystalloid is no longer recommended in the volume resuscitation of the trauma patient; it has even been demonstrated to worsen Systemic Inflammatory Response Syndrome (SIRS), Acute Respiratory Distress Syndrome (ARDS) and Multi Organ Failure (MOF), and blood and

Flowchart 3.1: Royal London Code Red Protocol.

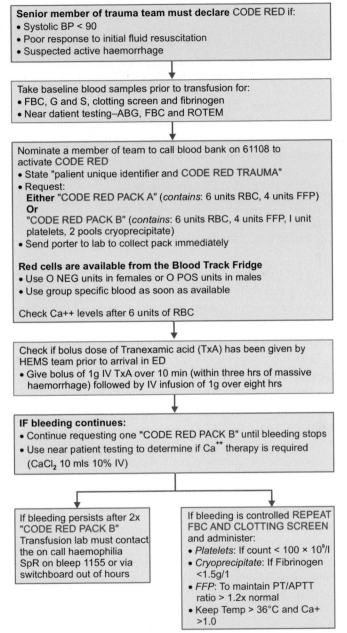

CODE RED TRAUMA–Massive haemorrhage

Senior member of trauma team must declare CODE RED if:
- Systolic BP < 90
- Poor response to initial fluid resuscitation
- Suspected active haemorrhage

Take baseline blood samples prior to transfusion for:
- FBC, G and S, clotting screen and fibrinogen
- Near datient testing–ABG, FBC and ROTEM

Nominate a member of team to call blood bank on 61108 to activate CODE RED
- State "palient unique identifier and CODE RED TRAUMA"
- Request:
  Either "CODE RED PACK A" (*contains*: 6 units RBC, 4 units FFP)
  Or
  "CODE RED PACK B" (*contains*: 6 units RBC, 4 units FFP, I unit platelets, 2 pools cryoprecipitate)
- Send porter to lab to collect pack immediately

Red cells are available from the Blood Track Fridge
- Use O NEG units in females or O POS units in males
- Use group specific blood as soon as available

Check Ca++ levels after 6 units of RBC

Check if bolus dose of Tranexamic acid (TxA) has been given by HEMS team prior to arrival in ED
- Give bolus of 1g IV TxA over 10 min (within three hrs of massive haemorrhage) followed by IV infusion of 1g over eight hrs

IF bleeding continues:
- Continue requesting one "CODE RED PACK B" until bleeding stops
- Use near patient testing to determine if Ca^{++} therapy is required ($CaCl_2$ 10 mls 10% IV)

If bleeding persists after 2x "CODE RED PACK B" Transfusion lab must contact the on call haemophilia SpR on bleep 1155 or via switchboard out of hours

If bleeding is controlled REPEAT FBC AND CLOTTING SCREEN and administer:
- *Platelets*: If count < 100 × 10⁹/l
- *Cryoprecipitate*: If Fibrinogen <1.5g/1
- *FFP*: To maintain PT/APTT ratio > 1.2x normal
- Keep Temp > 36°C and Ca+ >1.0

Source: Property of Barts Health NHS Trust.

blood products are the treatment of choice.[25] Agreed "massive haemorrhage" rather than "massive transfusion" protocols (Flowchart 3.1) can facilitate rapid mobilisation of pre-issued blood products, especially if the requisite products are stored in areas adjacent to the ED.

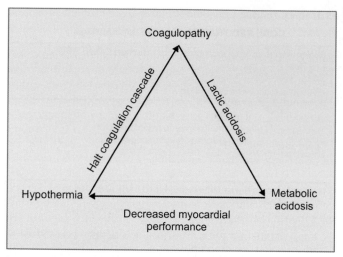

Fig. 3.4: The Lethal Triad of Death in Trauma Patients.
Source: www.wikepedia.org (trauma coagulopathy).

Initial DCR protocols emphasised early resuscitation of shocked patients with equivalent or near-equivalent ratios of blood and plasma with follow-on use of platelets and cryoprecipitate.[26] Recent advances in this approach have capitalised on the use of Rotational Elastometry or Thromboelastography (ROTEM) to provide near-real time, point-of-care data on the patient's clotting profile. Both techniques measure evolving clot strength as a function of time and can be utilised to diagnose whether poor clot strength is due to deficiency in factors, platelet function or hyperfibrinolysis, allowing a more bespoke transfusion intervention.[27] This potentially means earlier restoration of normal clotting, better physiological recovery and all the health and cost benefits associated with diminished use of blood and blood products.

A large, international multi-centre randomised study of use of tranexamic acid strongly points to the benefits of this cheap and well tolerated anti-fibrinolytic in reducing mortality if it is administered early, with no resultant increase in thromboembolic events.[8]

Appropriate DCR may diminish the requirement for DCS—in that a warm well-resuscitated patient may be able to tolerate a definitive surgical procedure at the first encounter rather than requiring an abbreviated procedure aimed at curtailing surgery that goes beyond control of bleeding and contamination.[28]

Key Point

- Shocked patients with stab injuries require timely blood and blood product therapy. Agreed massive haemorrhage protocols that facilitate rapid transfusion of blood should be understood by surgeons responsible for major trauma patients.

MANAGEMENT

The techniques of DCS are well described.[24,28,29] Interventional radiological options are infrequently applicable in penetrating trauma but include solid organ or deep muscle bed embolisation, in the case of active haemorrhage or pseudoaneurysm, and the deployment of covered stents for specific, discrete vascular injuries (e.g. subclavian artery). There have been major changes in the management of solid organ injury and there is now value in nonoperative management of penetrating injury to the liver, spleen and kidney.[30-32] Initially, the decision as to whether to operate or manage conservatively was based on both haemodynamic stability and grade of injury. However, based on large prospective trials, even in higher grade injuries, of liver, spleen and kidney, nonoperative management is appropriate in the haemodynamically stable patient, regardless of the grade of injury. This saves an unnecessary laparotomy in all patients, a high level of postoperative sepsis, blood transfusion and lifelong antibiotics in the event of splenectomy, and, of course, renal salvage which is preferable. It is paramount that the patient's vital signs are closely monitored, ideally in a high dependency unit. There is, of course, no role of nonoperative management of trauma to the gastrointestinal tract, as this can result in significant contamination. The primary concern with the conservative approach is the incidence of missed injuries, particularly to the bowel and pancreas, although cases of this remain low (2.3% in one series).[33] The conservative management of penetrating trauma (selective nonoperative management—SNOM) to the abdomen—where there is no evidence of haemodynamic instability or peritonitis—is therefore more established than was the case.[30-33] However, such strategies rely upon frequent, expert review, optimally by the same clinician, and a compliant, alert patient in order to pick up patients who subsequently fail their SNOM and require laparotomy.

Key Point

- A good grounding in DCS is invaluable for management of the shocked stab patient. In stable patients without evidence of peritonism SNOM offers an acceptable management plan although the patient must be scrupulously re-assessed.

INJURY PREVENTION

Trauma continues to be a major public health issue, in particularly, because it affects the young, working population of a community. Prevention of interpersonal violence, including knife crime, is a complex task, as a full understanding of deeper structural causes of inequalities within a community must be gleaned, and there is certainly no fast track method to achieve this.[34]

Key Point

- Trauma surgeons should involve themselves as much as possible with local injury prevention programmes.

Weapon carrying is multifactorial, associated with fear, aggression, coercion and expression strongly associated with socioeconomic status and often a "gang culture".[35] Attempts to theorise behaviours behind the use of weapons include individual and group dynamics, a motivation behind criminal behaviour, and how this translated to going through with an assault (Flowchart 3.2). These can go some way to understanding the root cause, and address target points along the pathway for prevention methods.[36]

Flowchart 3.2: Weapons and violence: A review of theory and research.

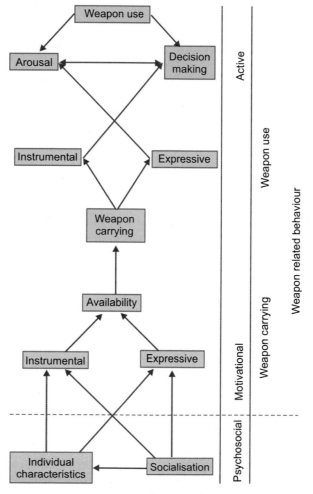

Source: With permission from Brennan IR, Moore SC. Weapons and violence: A review of theory and research. Aggression Violent Behavior. 2009;14(3):215-25.

Prevention strategies aim at either educating at-risk groups before criminal activity takes place, or preventing re-offending by providing psychosocial and community support. All of these have a cost benefit measure, both to the victim, offender and the taxpayer, and although there have been some studies in the United States conducted,[37] there is little comparative data from the United Kingdom. This is desperately required to enable resources to be deployed which are effective both in cost and effect.

CONCLUSION

Knife trauma remains a significant public health issue, however, improvement in outcomes is being seen as both pre-, and in hospital care is exponentially improving. The introduction of the major trauma centre network has been vitally important for improving outcomes following major trauma, meaning the right patients meet the right skilled clinicians and resources at the right time. Treatment of trauma patients is very much an integrated task with each spoke of the multidisciplinary team of equal value. Whilst is important that progress continues, there is a large deficiency in the investment in prevention strategies, and if clinicians engage more fully with these, then some gravitas can be placed on this important factor in the management of knife injuries.

REFERENCES

1. http://www.nationaltraumainstitute.org/home/trauma_statistics.html.
2. Mathers C, Ma Fat D, Boerma JT. The Global Burden of Disease: 2004 Update. World Health Organization; 2008.
3. Crewdson K, Weaver AE, Davies GE, et al. The incidence of penetrating trauma in London: have previously reported increases persisted in the last six years?. Scandinavian Journal of Trauma, Resuscitation and Emergency Medicine. 2014; 22(Suppl 1), P3.
4. Hodgetts TJ, Mahoney PF. Military pre-hospital care: why is it different? J R Army Med Corps. 2009;155(1):4-8.
5. Lockey DJ, Healey BA, Weaver AE, et al. Is there a requirement for advanced airway management for trauma patients in the pre-hospital phase of care? Scand J Trauma, Resusc Emerg Med. 2014;22(Suppl 1):P8.
6. Wang SY, Liao CH, Fu CY, et al. An outcome prediction model for exsanguinating patients with blunt abdominal trauma after damage control laparotomy: a retrospective study. BMC surgery 2014;14(1):24.
7. O'Reilly DJ, Morrison JJ, Jansen JO, et al. Prehospital blood transfusion in the en route management of severe combat trauma: a matched cohort study. Journal of Trauma and Acute Care Surgery. 2014;77(3),S114-S120.
8. Reade MC, Pitt V, Gruen RL. Tranexamic Acid and Trauma: Current Status and Knowledge Gaps with Recommended Research Priorities Shock 39 (2) & colon; 121–126, 2013. Shock, 2013;40(2):160-61.
9. Morrison JJ, Ross JD, Dubose JJ, et al. Military application of tranexamic acid in trauma emergency resuscitation (MATTERs) study. Arch Surg. 2012;147(2): 113-9.

10. Lamb CM, MacGoey P, Navarro AP, et al. Damage control surgery in the era of damage control resuscitation. British journal of anaesthesia. 2014;113(2): 242-49.
11. Davenport RA, Tai N, West A, et al. A major trauma centre is a specialty hospital not a hospital of specialties. Br J Surg. 2010;97(1):109-17.
12. Garwe T, Cowan LD, Neas BR et al, Directness of transport of major trauma patients to a level I trauma center: a propensity-adjusted survival analysis of the impact on short-term mortality. J Trauma Acute Care Surg. 2011;70(5):1118-27.
13. Davis JS, Sataloo SS, Butler FK, et al. An analysis of prehospital deaths: who can we save? J Trauma Acute Care Surg. 2014;77(2):213-8.
14. Radvinsky DS, Yoon RS, Schmitt PJ, et al. Evolution and development of the Advanced Trauma Life Support (ATLS) protocol: a historical perspective. Orthopedics. 2012;35(4):305-11.
15. Passos E, Dingley B, Smith A, et al. Tourniquet use for peripheral vascular injuries in the civilian setting. Injury. 2014;45(3):573-7.
16. Kragh JF Jr, O'Neil ML, Walters TJ, et al. Minor morbidity with emergency tourniquet use to stop bleeding in severe limb trauma: research, history, and reconciling advocates and abolitionists. Mil Med. 2011;176(7):817-23.
17. Pozza M, Millner RWJ. Celox (chitosan) for haemostasis in massive traumatic bleeding: experience in Afghanistan. Eur J Emerg Med. 2011;18(1):31-3.
18. Kuhls DA, Risucci DA, Bowyer MW, et al. Advanced surgical skills for exposure in trauma: a new surgical skills cadaver course for surgery residents and fellows. J Trauma Acute Care Surg. 2013;74(2):664-70.
19. Lockey DJ, Lyon RM, Davies GE. Development of a simple algorithm to guide the effective management of traumatic cardiac arrest. Resuscitation. 2013;84(6): 738-42.
20. Davies GE, Lockey DJ. Thirteen survivors of prehospital thoracotomy for penetrating trauma: a prehospital physician-performed resuscitation procedure that can yield good results. J Trauma Acute Care Surg. 2011;70(5):E75-8.
21. Moore EE, Knudson MM, Burlew CC, et al. Defining the limits of resuscitative emergency department thoracotomy: a contemporary Western Trauma Association perspective. J Trauma Acute Care Surg. 2011;70(2):334-9.
22. Huber-Wagner S, Lefering R, Qvick LM, et al. Effect of whole-body CT during trauma resuscitation on survival: a retrospective, multicentre study. The Lancet 2009;373(9673):1455-61.
23. Riskin DJ, Tsai TC, Loren-Riskin BS, et al. Massive transfusion protocols: the role of aggressive resuscitation versus product ratio in mortality reduction. J Am Coll Surg. 2009;209(2):198-205.
24. Davenport R, Manson J, De'Ath H, et al. Functional definition and characterisation of acute traumatic coagulopathy. Crit Care Med. 2011;39(12):2652-8.
25. Ertmer C, Kampmeier T, Rehberg S, et al. Fluid resuscitation in multiple trauma patients. Curr Opin Anesthesiol. 2011;24(2):202-8.
26. Davenport R, Curry N, Manson J et al. Hemostatic effects of fresh frozen plasma may be maximal at red cell ratios of 1: 2. J Trauma Acute Care Surg. 2011;70(1):90-6.
27. Woolley T, Midwinter M, Spencer P, et al. Utility of interim ROTEM values of clot strength, A5 and A10, in predicting final assessment of coagulation status in severely injured battle patients. Injury. 2013;44(5):593-9.
28. Schreiber MA. The beginning of the end for damage control surgery. Br J Surg. 2012;99(S1):10-1.

29. Cirocchi R, Abraha I, Montedori A, et al. Damage control surgery for abdominal trauma. Cochrane Database Syst Rev. 2010;1:p2-9
30. Como JJ, Bokhari F, Chiu WC et al. Practice management guidelines for selective nonoperative management of penetrating abdominal trauma. J Trauma Acute Care Surg. 2010; 68(3):721-33.
31. Hope WW, Smith ST, Medieros B, et al. Non-operative management in penetrating abdominal trauma: is it feasible at a Level II trauma center? J Emerg Med. 2012;43(1):190-5.
32. Jansen JO, Inaba K, Rizoli SB, et al. Selective non-operative management of penetrating abdominal injury in Great Britain and Ireland: survey of practice. Injury. 2012;43(11):1799-1804.
33. Miller PR, Croce MA, Bee TK, et al. Associated injuries in blunt solid organ trauma: implications for missed injury in nonoperative management. J Trauma Injury, Inf, Crit Care. 2002;53(2):238-44.
34. Eades C. Knife Crime: Ineffective Reactions to a Distracting Problem? A Review of Evidence and Policy. London: The Centre for Crime and Justice Studies; 2006.
35. Brennan IR, Moore SC. Weapons and violence: a review of theory and research. Aggress Violent Beh. 2009;14(3):215-25.
36. Webb E, Wyatt JP, Henry T, et al. A comparison of fatal with non-fatal knife injuries in Edinburgh. Forensic Sci Int. 1999;99(3):179-87.
37. Drake EK, Aos S, Miller MG. Evidence-based public policy options to reduce crime and criminal justice costs: implications in Washington State. Victims Offenders. 2009;4:170-96.

4

Chapter

An Update on Intravenous Fluids in Surgical Practice

Mike Stroud

INTRODUCTION

Decisions on intravenous (IV) fluid and electrolyte provision for surgical patients are often difficult yet usually delegated to junior doctors who lack relevant experience and specific training. In their recent 2013 guidance, NICE (National Institute for Health and Care Excellence) reported surveys that show the majority of IV fluid prescribers know neither the normal fluid and electrolyte needs of patients nor the specific composition of available fluids.[1] It is not therefore surprising that inappropriate IV fluids were identified as a significant contributor to morbidity and mortality in a UK National Confidential Enquiry into Perioperative Deaths[2] and although that report recommended making IV fluid prescribing equal in status to drug prescribing, this did not happen. Even if rarely reported, both inadequate and excessive IV fluids and/or electrolyte provision almost certainly continue to generate complications, prolonged hospital stay and increased cost.[1-7]

Poor IV fluid practice in surgery probably occurs more frequently in emergency departments, acute admission units and general wards than in operating theatres and intensive care. The 2013 NICE recommendations therefore concentrate on fluid prescribing for general settings, and this chapter has a similar focus. NICE also recognised that best fluid prescriptions were extremely variable and not really amenable to proscriptive rules. Their most important recommendations therefore revolve around the need for all IV fluid prescribers to understand the principles of fluid balance in health and disease and for all hospitals to organize appropriate training and to monitor adverse, IV fluid-related events.

PROBLEMS OF PRESCRIBING IV FLUIDS IN SURGERY

The aims of IV fluid therapy are to ensure that total fluid and electrolyte requirements are met and existing abnormalities are corrected if possible in patients where this cannot be achieved by oral or enteral routes. There are many reasons why providing optimal IV fluids is difficult in surgical cases, especially in ward type settings with less intensive monitoring. Reasonably detailed description of these problems can be found in the full

NICE guidance,[1] and they are also covered in the NICE IV fluid training tool found at http://elearning.nice.org.uk/login/index.php. However, they are summarized below.

1. *Lack of evidence*:

   The evidence to determine best practice in general surgical settings is limited because:

   a. Many accepted IV fluid practices are based on historical, practical, production issues rather than randomised controlled trials (RCTs).

   b. IV fluid studies cannot easily be pooled for meta-analysis as they examine variable outcomes in heterogeneous groups using not only different types of fluid with differing electrolyte content but different volumes and rates of administration, sometimes with additional inotrope use.

   c. Most published RCTs were undertaken in intensive care or intraoperative settings, which particularly limit interpretation of best fluids for resuscitation as comparisons of different fluid types are made either after actual initial resuscitation has taken place (randomization occurs once patients have reached critical care) or are made in patients with anaesthesia-induced hypovolaemia—a situation, which does not closely mirror other causes of circulatory collapse.

2. *Problems with salt and water overload*:

   There are many reasons why surgical patients are prone to salt and water overload, particularly in the early postoperative phase:

   a. Humans have powerful sodium retention mechanisms regulated largely by renin–angiotensin (the kidney can reduce urinary Na+ concentration to < 5 mmol/L), but our capacity to excrete excess sodium is poor, probably because we evolved in the hot, low-sodium environment of Africa where excess natural intake would never occur. Illness or injury, particularly major surgery, further enhances sodium retention due to increases in antidiuretic hormone and cortisol as well as renin-triggered aldosterone, and simultaneously, the capacity to excrete excess sodium is markedly impaired.

   b. Perioperative responses increase the transcapillary albumin loss by up to 300% from about 5%/hour in health to 13–15%/hour[8] and subsequent falls in plasma albumin then reduce intravascular volume (with further stimulation of renin), whilst increased interstitial albumin promotes oedema.

   c. Many surgical patients start their postoperative course in very positive sodium and water balance because of high intraoperative IV fluid provision needed to compensate for anaesthetic-induced vasodilatation.

   d. Even healthy kidneys can only excrete a limited solute load—a capacity easily overwhelmed by catabolic release of solutes that is added to any iatrogenic solute excess.[9]

e. 0.9% saline, containing 154-mmol/L sodium, is widely used despite the fact that normal maintenance needs are only 1 mmol/kg/day, which would be met in most cases by only 0.5 L of the fluid.

f. The intense sodium and water retentive responses described above imply that some postoperative oliguria is normal[10] and hence the common practice of meeting any degree of oliguria with a "give more fluids" reflex often worsens salt and water overload. Additional IV fluids should only be given if there are signs of intravascular volume deficit.

g. Since water as well as sodium is retained postoperatively, surgical patients easily develop dilutional hyponatraemia when given excess glucose or glucose/saline. This then encourages provision of 0.9% saline despite the fact that many hyponatraemic patients are oedematous with high total body sodium. Postoperative hyponatraemia is therefore best prevented or managed by decreasing total fluid provision rather than giving more sodium although this does not apply in some surgical cases where there are high, abnormal sodium losses (*see* below).

h. Potassium depletion is a poorly recognised cause of additional sodium retention. In the presence of deficiency, H+ ion reabsorption is impaired causing hypokalaemic alkalosis and decreased capacity to excrete sodium. Depletion of potassium is common in postoperative situations because the activation of aldosterone precipitates high urinary loss and the catabolic release of negatively charged intracellular amino acids causes simultaneous leakage of positively charged intracellular potassium ions. When catabolism is extreme, the latter process can lead to hyperkalaemia, especially if renal function is impaired, but in many postoperative patients, especially those with additional gastrointestinal (GI) tract potassium loss, hypokalaemia or at least whole body potassium depletion does occur and needs correction to help treat sodium and water excess.

i. Malnutrition is common in surgical patients and is often accompanied by reductions in cell membrane pumping with consequent movement of sodium and water into cells and simultaneous movement of potassium, magnesium, calcium and phosphate out which are then lost in the urine. Malnourished individuals therefore tend to have high total body sodium and water with low total body potassium, phosphate and magnesium (even if plasma levels are normal). This makes them even more prone to salt and water overload.

j. Malnourished patients are also vulnerable to refeeding syndrome with the delivery of IV glucose or food promoting insulin release, which not only stimulates cellular glucose uptake but reactivates the cell membrane pumps. This then leads plasma potassium, phosphate and magnesium moving back into cells with simultaneous movement of sodium and water back out into the circulation, effectively adding to any IV salt and water provision.[11] Furthermore, malnourished patients often have diminished cardiac and renal reserve and/or hidden infection with high capillary escape rates. Advice on the prevention and management of refeeding syndrome can be found in NICE guidance on Nutrition Support REF.

k. Although it is well recognized that hyperchloraemia can cause hyperchloraemic acidosis, the fact that high plasma chloride promotes ileus[12] and markedly reduces renal perfusion and glomerular filtration is less well known.[13] Administration of IV fluids with high chloride content must clearly predispose individuals to this although conversely, inadequate IV provision of chloride in patients with high GI salt losses can cause hypochloraemic alkalosis. Since 0.9% sodium chloride contains 154 mmol/L of chloride and normal plasma levels are only 95–105 mmol/L, prolonged saline use may also promote oedematous states and temporary intestinal failure via hyperchloraemia as well as other mechanisms.

3. *Problems in making accurate allowance for abnormal fluid and electrolyte losses*:

Many surgical patients have significant external losses of fluid and electrolytes, often from the GI or urinary tracts although high losses also occur with fever and burns. The presence of existing deficits from these losses and/or ongoing abnormal loss creates many problems for IV fluid prescribing:

a. The losses are usually difficult to measure in terms of both volume and electrolyte content.

b. High GI sodium loss is common, potentially causing hyponatraemia from total body sodium depletion. This must be distinguished from the hyponatraemia caused by excess low sodium fluid in patients with activated salt and water retention when total body sodium is high. In truly sodium depleted cases, proper assessment of likely sodium balance will often confirm high likely losses, e.g. from a high output, high GI stoma, coupled with clearly inadequate provision, and spot urinary measurement will usually shows very low sodium levels. However, spot urinary measures can only be interpreted if renal function is reasonable and the use of diuretics also confuses the picture.

c. Any deficits, which developed slowly, can be accompanied by compensatory adaptations and so must only be reversed slowly to limit risks of problems such as pontine demyelinosis.

4. *Problems from internal fluid redistribution*:

In addition to abnormal external losses, many surgical patients have marked internal fluid and electrolyte distribution changes especially after major interventions, when septic or critically ill, or with significant comorbidities. Most develop high transcapillary escape and whole body sodium and water excess with pulmonary and peripheral oedema, weight gain, compartment syndrome and poor wound healing, coupled with low intravascular volumes and renal dysfunction. IV fluid prescribing in such cases is not surprisingly extremely difficult.

5. *Problems of organ dysfunction*:

Many surgical patients have specific organ or system dysfunction related to: their primary surgical problem; complications such as shock, sepsis or drug reactions or existing comorbidities. Cardiac, renal or hepatic dysfunction particularly increases vulnerability to salt and water overload.

6. *Problems of poor record keeping*:

Even though regular, accurate monitoring of all relevant parameters must be considered as a standard of care for surgical patients on IV fluids, current measurement and recording of fluid and electrolyte inputs (especially those contained in other IV drugs) are often poor, as are recordings and summary additions of outputs from all sources. Accurate documentation of sequential weight, which is incredibly valuable in making optimal fluid provision choices, is rarely done well although it must be recognised that even with modern equipment, accurate weight measurement may be impractical in immobile patients with drains, etc. and interpretation of sequential weight is subject to many confounders including fluid loss into drains and dressings and the redistribution of fluid as oedema or fluid in non-functioning gut or natural body cavities.

Key Points

- The evidence to determine best practice in general surgical settings is limited.
- Many surgical patients have significant external losses of fluid and electrolytes, often from the GI or urinary tracts although high losses also occur with fever and burns.
- Surgical patients are prone to salt and water overload, particularly in the early postoperative phase.

ASSESSMENT OF IV FLUID AND ELECTROLYTE NEEDS IN SURGICAL PATIENTS

Any patient requiring IV fluids needs assessment revolving round 4 indications for fluids, which NICE designated as the "4Rs" and incorporated into prescribing algorithms along with a 5th R for reassessment (Flowchart 4.1). The algorithms that also include some guidance on volumes and types of fluid to use based on evidence discussed in the "Choice of fluid type" section below. The 4Rs are:

1. Resuscitation—Some surgical patients have rapid external losses of circulatory volume from bleeding, drains, plasma loss or the GI tract whilst others have high internal loss to the extravascular space or internal body compartments. Urgent fluid resuscitation and other measures are needed if acute or chronic fluid loss has led to circulatory decompensation often accompanied by specific system dysfunction especially of the central nervous system with agitation, confusion or decreased consciousness or cardiac arrhythmias and renal dysfunction. There is, however, a problem in that fluid overload also precipitates most of the same symptoms and signs so inexperienced doctors may mistake overload for depletion. Furthermore, there is wide variability in patients' underlying fitness and those with significant comorbidities may decompensate with relatively little fluid depletion whilst the young, in particular, may maintain systolic blood pressure until suddenly severe shock ensues.

2. Routine maintenance—Advances in surgery, anaesthesia and perioperative care have reduced the period of postoperative GI dysfunction and early removal of nasogastric drains and commencement of reasonable oral intake is now the norm. The routine use of postoperative IV maintenance fluids has therefore declined and the consequent reduction in iatrogenic salt and water overload may well be an under recognised contributor to the success of early rehabilitation after surgery protocols. Nevertheless, many surgical patients still need IV fluids pre- or postoperatively for essentially routine maintenance purposes and prescribing for those with more complex fluid and electrolyte issues, needs to start with estimates of routine maintenance needs appropriate to body weight followed by adjustments either up or down.

3. Replacement—As discussed above, many surgical patients need additional IV fluids to treat previous and/or ongoing abnormal losses.

4. Redistribution—As also discussed above, many surgical patients have marked internal fluid distribution changes.

The "4Rs" approach demands careful, individual patient assessment by competent clinicians using all available information including: a focussed history; brief general examination with specific assessment of fluid status from trends in pulse and blood pressure, JVP and presence of oedema, and review of fluid balance and body weight charts. Recent laboratory results and trends are also needed.

Once an estimate of total fluid volume and electrolytes requirements has been made, a common prescribing error is to fail to allow for fluid and electrolyte intakes from all other sources. These may include oral or enteral tube provision as well as any other IV therapies. Blood products, in particular, contain large amounts of electrolytes as do many IV drugs, especially when given frequently in large volume diluents, e.g. the sodium content of some IV antibiotics easily exceeds daily sodium needs. Most patients on artificial

Flowchart 4.1: National Institute for Health and Care Excellence algorithms for intravenous fluid therapy.

Algorithms for IV fluid therapy

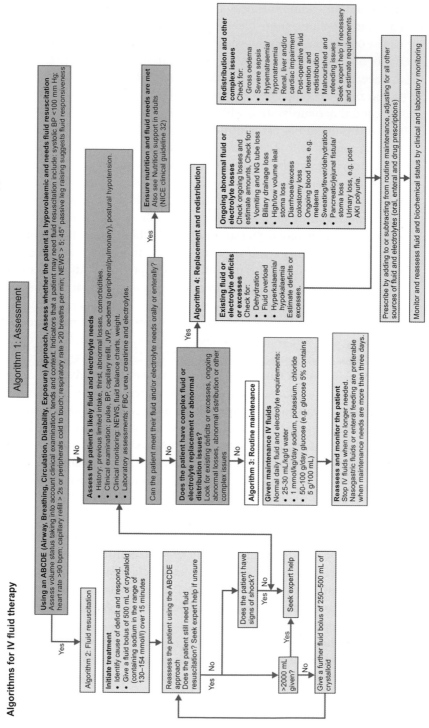

nutrition also receive adequate fluid and electrolytes to meet at least their routine maintenance needs, yet prescription of inappropriate additional IV fluids is frequent.

REASSESSMENT AND MONITORING

Even when taking a structured "4Rs" approach, estimates of IV fluid and electrolyte need will often prove incorrect, especially as clinical states are usually changing. There is therefore a need for constant clinical and laboratory. *Reassessment* (the 5th R) with regimens altered or stopped as appropriate. This should initially include at least daily reassessments of clinical fluid status and fluid balance charts and weight measurement twice weekly if at all possible. In complex or vulnerable patients, clinical reassessment will need to be even more frequent.

Laboratory monitoring of urea, creatinine and electrolytes is also needed daily during initial IV fluid therapy and, as noted above, additional intermittent monitoring of urinary sodium may be helpful. Chloride should also be measured in patients receiving significant amounts of high chloride (>120 mmol/L) fluids (*see* discussions below).

Importantly, the need for continuing IV fluids is not always questioned by junior trainees who may be inclined simply to repeat previous days' IV fluid prescriptions rather than properly reassess patients. They should therefore be encouraged to seek advice from more senior colleagues and proper review of IV fluids *must* be an integral part of every surgical ward round.

Key Point

- Any patient requiring IV fluids needs assessment revolving round 4 indications for fluids, which NICE designated as the "4Rs" resuscitation, routine maintenance, replacement and redistribution. A "5th R" reassessment and monitoring is also essential.

CHOICE OF IV FLUID TYPE

The problems of inadequate RCT evidence mentioned above have led to much debate about the best regimens to use for resuscitation and routine maintenance, and since there are virtually no RCTs relevant to best replacement and redistribution issues, there is also uncertainty when prescribing for those indications.

The Best Regimens for Resuscitation

A variety of crystalloids, artificial colloids and human albumin solutions have been used for fluid resuscitation. Although traditional teaching suggested colloids had advantages, the idea that they are much better at expanding and maintaining intravascular volume is now doubted and they are much more expensive than crystalloids. Although in theory, colloids that are iso-oncotic with plasma should expand blood volume by the volume infused, in practice the figure is closer to 60–80%[14,15] and probably much less in sick patients with high transcapillary leakage. Furthermore, studies showing that circulatory stability is better maintained by colloid rather than crystalloid in anaesthetic-induced hypovolaemia may not be relevant to ward patients with illness/injury-induced hypovolaemia and abnormal fluid distribution and handling.

Any advantage of colloids are also offset by potential problems of renal dysfunction, disturbed coagulation and allergic responses and since nearly all currently available semi-synthetic colloids contain 140–154 mmol/L sodium chloride, their use may also contribute to excess sodium and chloride provision.

In the United Kingdom sodium chloride 0.9%, Ringer's lactate/acetate, Hartmann's solution, gelatins, hydroxyethyl starch, and albumin are all used for resuscitation in general surgical areas whilst the use of dextrans or high molecular weight penta- and hexa starches is usually confined to intraoperative and ICU usage. NICE therefore only evaluated studies comparing those used in general areas to each other. The evaluations showed:

Key Points

- Gelatins had no clear advantage over other colloids or crystalloids.[15-22]
- Tetrastarch had no clear advantage over other colloids or crystalloids,[23-27] and three large studies in critical care suggested it may increase acute kidney injury (AKI) compared to 0.9% saline or Ringer's lactate with one suggesting increased mortality.
- Albumin 4% had no clear advantage compared to 0.9% saline although there was a trend towards decreased mortality in one study examining its use in a pre-defined sepsis subgroup.[28,29]
- No studies compared colloids made up in balanced physiological solutions to those made up in sodium chloride 0.9%.
- Studies of factors such as timing, administration rates and best total volume of fluids to give for resuscitation[30-34] showed apparently important differences between early versus late, and fast versus slow fluid provision but the direction of benefit was not always the same in different studies.

The NICE concluded that crystalloids containing sodium in the range 130–154 mmol/L should be used for resuscitation rather than colloids and that an initial bolus of 500 mL should be given over < 15 minutes. They also recommended that tetrastarches should no longer be used and that albumin could be considered severe sepsis although in reality, the cost implications of this will surely confine its use to experts in critical or high-care settings.

The Best Regimen for Routine Maintenance

Sodium chloride 0.9% with or without additional potassium is the most commonly used IV fluid in UK surgical patients, but it may contribute to excessive sodium and water retention. There is therefore interest in "balanced fluids", which contain less sodium and chloride and variable amounts of potassium, calcium and magnesium at levels approximating to normal needs.

Five per cent glucose and glucose/salines with or without potassium cannot be used for rapid administration but once the glucose is metabolised, they are distributed through total body water with limited effects on blood volume. They are therefore appropriate for preventing or correcting simple dehydration and also help limit starvation ketosis, although they make little contribution to meeting patients' overall nutritional needs.

The NICE found no studies that simply compared different maintenance fluid choices to one another but four RCTs[35-38] compared "restricted" IV fluid maintenance regimens (with reduced sodium chloride and fluid volumes) with more "standard" regimens in postoperative patients. Two RCTs suggested that restricted regimens reduced mortality and hospital stays whilst the other two showed no difference in mortality with one suggesting restricted regimens prolonged hospital stays. However, the four studies varied enormously with restricted groups given fluid volumes ranging from 1.5–2.5 L/day with sodium chloride provision ranging from 62–231 mmol/day, whereas the standard regimen groups received fluid volumes of 2–4 L/day with sodium chloride provision ranging from 154–231 mmol/day. This not only prevented meaningful meta-analysis but probably explains the differences in results with adverse outcomes seen if either too much or too little fluid and too much or too little sodium chloride is given. Importantly, all four RCTs suggested no clinically important difference in the risks of developing AKI when using restricted IV fluid regimens and none reported significant problems of hyponatraemia even though sodium chloride provision was at low levels that have traditionally been thought of as likely to precipitate hyponatraemic risks.

The NICE also reviewed studies in which surgical patients received IV fluids with chloride >120 mmol/L with those receiving fluids with chloride < 120 mmol/L[1] and concluded that provision of lower chloride fluids was probably associated with lower mortality and morbidity. In a separate review of studies examining associations between serum chloride input, plasma levels and clinical outcome[1] suggested that hyperchloraemia occurred more frequently if high chloride fluids were given but that both hyper- and hypo-chloraemia had adverse outcome effects. These considerations led to NICE recommending that serum chloride should initially be monitored daily when using regimens based on fluids containing >120 mmol/L chloride and that if chloride levels rise, hyperchloraemic acidosis should be considered. Low chloride levels are most likely to reflect true saline depletion.

The conclusion of all of the above findings was a NICE recommendation that for routine maintenance an appropriate initial prescription should deliver approximately: 25–30 mL/kg/day of water; 1 mmol/kg/day of potassium, sodium and chloride; and 50–100 g/day of glucose. NICE also suggested that this could be achieved by using 25–30 mL/kg/day of sodium chloride 0.18% in 4% glucose with 27 mmol/L potassium—a fluid that became very unpopular with surgeons because of its association with hyponatraemia. However, NICE felt that hyponatraemic risks were small if <2.5 L/day is used and explicitly pointed out that these were only initial prescriptions with further prescribing needing to be guided by monitoring. They also recommended that less fluid (e.g. 20–25 mL/kg/day) should be considered in patients who are older or frail and those with renal impairment, cardiac failure or malnutrition.

The Best Fluid for Replacement

If patients need IV fluids and electrolytes for replacement purposes, it is important to recognize that these will usually be in addition to their routine maintenance requirements. Replacement for blood loss is generally by the use of 0.9% sodium chloride or balanced crystalloids with packed red cells as necessary, whilst replacement for other losses, e.g. GI or urinary, will usually depend on estimates of their composition but 0.9% sodium chloride, glucose 5% and glucose with saline solutions and balanced crystalloids can all be used with or without additional potassium as appropriate. Although it is sometimes possible to measure the volumes and electrolyte content of abnormal losses (e.g. with high urinary loss), more often it is only possible to measure volumes and not infrequently both volume and likely content must be estimated, predicting likely electrolyte losses from the nature of the loss (Fig. 4.1). Since these estimates will be subject to wide errors, particularly close clinical and laboratory monitoring will be needed.

The Best Fluids for Fluid Redistribution Problems

Prescribing appropriate IV fluids for patients with redistribution type problems is particularly difficult since too little leads to intravascular hypovolaemia, low blood pressure, poor urine output and poor tissue perfusion, whilst too much may promote even more oedema. Furthermore, as such patients get better, transcapillary leakage will decrease and the redistribution problems may effectively operate in reverse. It may therefore important to reduce overall IV fluid and electrolyte provision to permit a net negative sodium and water balance, to aid oedema resolution.

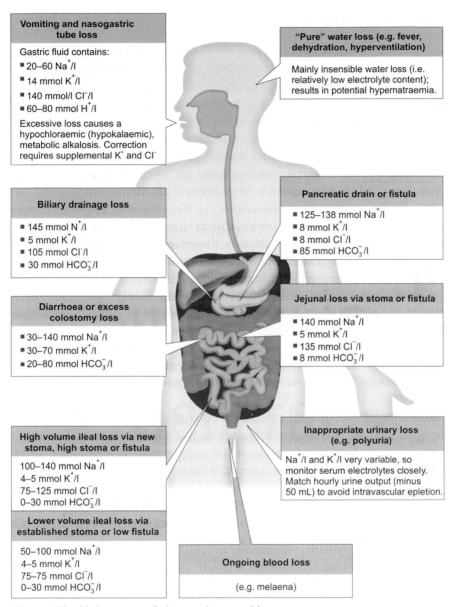

Vomiting and nasogastric tube loss

Gastric fluid contains:

- 20–60 Na^+/l
- 14 mmol K^+/l
- 140 mmol/l Cl^-/l
- 60–80 mmol H^+/l

Excessive loss causes a hypochloraemic (hypokalaemic), metabolic alkalosis. Correction requires supplemental K^+ and Cl^-

"Pure" water loss (e.g. fever, dehydration, hyperventilation)

Mainly insensible water loss (i.e. relatively low electrolyte content); results in potential hypernatraemia.

Biliary drainage loss

- 145 mmol N^+/l
- 5 mmol K^+/l
- 105 mmol Cl^-/l
- 30 mmol HCO_3^-/l

Pancreatic drain or fistula

- 125–138 mmol Na^+/l
- 8 mmol K^+/l
- 8 mmol Cl^-/l
- 85 mmol HCO_3^-/l

Diarrhoea or excess colostomy loss

- 30–140 mmol Na^+/l
- 30–70 mmol K^+/l
- 20–80 mmol HCO_3^-/l

Jejunal loss via stoma or fistula

- 140 mmol Na^+/l
- 5 mmol K^+/l
- 135 mmol Cl^-/l
- 8 mmol HCO_3^-/l

High volume ileal loss via new stoma, high stoma or fistula

100–140 mmol Na^+/l
4–5 mmol K^+/l
75–125 mmol Cl^-/l
0–30 mmol HCO_3^-/l

Lower volume ileal loss via established stoma or low fistula

50–100 mmol Na^+/l
4–5 mmol K^+/l
75–75 mmol Cl^-/l
0–30 mmol HCO_3^-/l

Inappropriate urinary loss (e.g. polyuria)

Na^+/l and K^+/l very variable, so monitor serum electrolytes closely. Match hourly urine output (minus 50 mL) to avoid intravascular epletion.

Ongoing blood loss

(e.g. melaena)

Fig. 4.1: The likely nature of abnormal external losses.
Source: Copyright-National Clinical Guideline Centre.

The overall approach is to treat intravascular hypovolaemia as one would for resuscitation but aim for a negative overall fluid and sodium balance as soon as possible. In severe cases, balance can be assessed by comparing total sodium intake (accounting for all sources including other IV fluids, IV drugs and their diluents) with total losses from urinary measurements and estimates of sodium in other external losses. Excretion should exceed intake.

A variety of IV fluid types are used in patients with internal redistribution issues including crystalloids, synthetic colloids and albumin. As discussed above, it seems likely that the use 0.9% sodium chloride will promote more sodium and water retention than balanced solutions, but NICE found no studies that made any comparisons of fluid types in this situation. Concentrated (20–25%) sodium poor albumin has been used for oedematous patients with a plasma volume deficit, aiming to draw fluid from the interstitial space and promote renal perfusion and excretion of sodium and water excess. However, this use is highly specialized and of uncertain benefit. Albumin is also used in some patients with hepatic failure and ascites, although its use in this setting is beyond the scope of this chapter.

As noted above, it is also important to correct potassium depletion to maximize sodium exchange, bearing in mind that plasma potassium is a poor marker of whole body status since it is primarily intracellular. However, if giving generous potassium, careful monitoring for hyperkalaemia is needed. Hyperchloraemia should also be avoided.[13]

Diuretics should only be used with caution since they may reduce circulating blood volume and consideration should always be given as to whether the same net effect on fluid balance might not be achieved through reduction of IV fluids, particularly a reduction in the provision of 0.9% sodium chloride. Twice weekly weighing, when possible, in addition to routine daily clinical examination allows oedema mobilization to be assessed.

Key Point

- Hospitals should establish systems to ensure that all health-care professionals involved in prescribing and delivering IV fluids are properly trained and clear incidents of fluid mismanagement (for example, unnecessarily prolonged dehydration or inadvertent iatrogenic fluid overload) should be reported through standard critical incident reporting, to enhance learning and experience.

REFERENCES

1. NICE guideline CG 174, IV Fluid therapy in adults in hospital. 2013. Available from www.nice.org.uk/guidance/cg174.
2. National Confidential Enquiry into Perioperative Deaths. Extremes of age: the 1999 report of the National Confidential Enquiry into Perioperative Deaths, 1999. [online] Available from: http://www.ncepod.org.uk/pdf/1999/99full.pdf.
3. Arieff AI. Fatal postoperative pulmonary edema: pathogenesis and literature review. Chest. 1999; 115(5):1371-7.
4. Herrod PJJ, Awad S, Redfern A, et al. Hypo- and hypernatraemia in surgical patients: is there room for improvement? World J Surg. 2010;34(3): 495-9.
5. Stoneham MD, Hill EL. Variability in post-operative fluid and electrolyte prescription. Br J Clin Pract. 1997;51(2):82-4.
6. Walsh SR, Cook EJ, Bentley R, et al. Perioperative fluid management: prospective audit. Int J Clin Pract. 2008;62(3):492-7.

7. Walsh SR, Walsh CJ. Intravenous fluid-associated morbidity in postoperative patients. Ann Royal College SurgEngl. 2005;87(2):126-30.
8. Fleck A, Raines G, Hawker F, et al. Increased vascular permeability: a major cause of hypoalbuminaemia in disease and injury. Lancet. 1985;1(8432):781-4.
9. Lobo DN. Fluid overload and surgical outcome: another piece in the jigsaw. Ann Surg. 2009;249(2):186-8.
10. Tindall SF, Clark RG. The influence of high and low sodium intakes on post-operative antidiuresis. Br J Surg. 1981;68(9):639-44.
11. Stanga Z, Brunner A, Leuenberger M, et al. Nutrition in clinical practice-the refeeding syndrome: illustrative cases and guidelines for prevention and treatment. Eur J Clin Nutr. 2008;62(6):687-94.
12. Lobo DN, Stanga Z, Simpson JA, et al. Dilution and redistribution effects of rapid 2-litre infusions of 0.9% (w/v) saline and 5% (w/v) dextrose on haematological parameters and serum biochemistry in normal subjects: a double-blind crossover study. Clin Sci. 2001;101(2):173-9.
13. Chowdhury AH, Cox EF, Francis ST, et al. A randomized, controlled, double-blind crossover study on the effects of 2-L infusions of 0.9% saline and plasma-lyte(R) 148 on renal blood flow velocity and renal cortical tissue perfusion in healthy volunteers. Ann Surg. 2012; 256(1):18-24.
14. Awad S, Dharmavaram S, Wearn CS, et al. Effects of an intraoperative infusion of 4% succinylated gelatine (Gelofusine(R)) and 6% hydroxyethyl starch (Voluven(R)) on blood volume. Br J Anaesth. 2012;109(2):168-76.
15. Lobo DN, Stanga Z, Aloysius MM, et al. Effect of volume loading with 1 liter intravenous infusions of 0.9% saline, 4% succinylated gelatine (Gelofusine) and 6% hydroxyethyl starch (Voluven) on blood volume and endocrine responses: a randomized, three-way crossover study in healthy volunteers. Crit Care Med. 2010;38(2):464-70.
16. Godet G, Lehot JJ, Janvier G, et al. Safety of HES 130/0.4 (Voluven(R)) in patients with preoperative renal dysfunction undergoing abdominal aortic surgery: a prospective, randomized, controlled, parallel-group multicentre trial. Eur J Anaesth Engl. 2008;25(12):986-94.
17. Gondos T, Marjanek Z, Ulakcsai Z, et al. Short-term effectiveness of different volume replacement therapies in postoperative hypovolaemic patients. Eur J Anaesth. 2010;27(9):794-800.
18. Innerhofer P, Fries D, Margreiter J, et al. The effects of perioperatively administered colloids and crystalloids on primary platelet-mediated hemostasis and clot formation. Anesth Anal. 2002;95(4):858-65.
19. Jin SL, Yu BW. Effects of acute hypervolemic fluid infusion of hydroxyethyl starch and gelatin on hemostasis and possible mechanisms. Clin Appl Thromb Hemost. 2010;16(1):91-8.
20. Mahmood A, Gosling P, Barclay R, et al. Splanchnic microcirculation protection by hydroxyethyl starches during abdominal aortic aneurysm surgery. Eur J Vasc Endovasc Surg. 2009;37(3):319-25.
21. Verheij J, van Lingen A, Beishuizen A, et al. Cardiac response is greater for colloid than saline fluid loading after cardiac or vascular surgery. Intensive Care Medicine. 2006;32(7):1030-8.
22. Wu JJ, Huang MS, Tang GJ, et al. Hemodynamic response of modified fluid gelatin compared with lactated ringer's solution for volume expansion in emergency resuscitation of hypovolemic shock patients: preliminary report of a prospective, randomized trial. World J Surg. 2001;25(5): 598-602.

23. Dubin A, Pozo MO, Casabella CA, et al. Comparison of 6% hydroxyethyl starch 130/0.4 and saline solution for resuscitation of the microcirculation during the early goal-directed therapy of septic patients. J Crit Care. 2010;25(4):659-8.

24. Guidet B, Martinet O, Boulain T, et al. Assessment of hemodynamic efficacy and safety of 6% hydroxyethylstarch 130/0.4 vs. 0.9% NaCl fluid replacement in patients with severe sepsis: the CRYSTMAS study. Crit Care. 2012;16(3):R94.

25. James MF, Michell WL, Joubert IA, et al. Resuscitation with hydroxyethyl starch improves renal function and lactate clearance in penetrating trauma in a randomized controlled study: the FIRST trial (Fluids in Resuscitation of Severe Trauma). Br J Anaesth. 2011;107(5):693-702.

26. Myburgh JA, Finfer S, Bellomo R, et al. Hydroxyethyl starch or saline for fluid resuscitation in intensive care. N Engl J Med. 2012; 367(20):1901-11.

27. Perner A, Haase N, Guttormsen AB, et al. Hydroxyethyl starch 130/0.42 versus Ringer's acetate in severe sepsis. N Engl J Med. 2012;367(2):124-34.

28. Roberts I, Blackhall K, Alderson P, et al. Human albumin solution for resuscitation and volume expansion in critically ill patients. Cochrane Database Syst Rev. 2011;(11):CD001208. DOI:10.1002/14651858.CD001208.pub4.

29. Guidet B, Mosqueda GJ, Priol G, et al. The COASST study: cost-effectiveness of albumin in severe sepsis and septic shock. J Crit Care. 2007;22(3):197-203.

30. Dutton RP, Mackenzie CF, Scalea TM. Hypotensive resuscitation during active hemorrhage: impact on in-hospital mortality. J Trauma—Injury Infection & Critical Care. 2002;52(6):1141-6.

31. Lin SM, Huang CD, Lin HC, et al. A modified goal-directed protocol improves clinical outcomes in intensive care unit patients with septic shock: a randomized controlled trial. Shock. 2006;26(6):551-7.

32. Mao Eq, Tang Yq, Fei J, et al. Fluid therapy for severe acute pancreatitis in acute response stage. Chin Med J. 2009;122(2):169-73.

33. Rivers E, Nguyen B, Havstad S, et al. Early goal-directed therapy in the treatment of severe sepsis and septic shock. N Engl J Med. 2001;345(19):1368-77.

34. Wiedemann HP, Wheeler AP, Bernard GR, et al. Comparison of two fluid-management strategies in acute lung injury. N Engl J Med. 2006;354(24):2564-75.

35. Gonzalez-Fajardo JA, Mengibar L, Brizuela JA, et al. Effect of postoperative restrictive fluid therapy in the recovery of patients with abdominal vascular surgery. Eur J Vasc Endovasc Surg. 2009;37(5):538-43.

36. Lobo DN, Bostock KA, Neal KR, et al. Effect of salt and water balance on recovery of gastrointestinal function after elective colonic resection: a randomised controlled trial. Lancet. 2002; 359(9320):1812-8.

37. MacKay G, Fearon K, McConnachie A, et al. Randomized clinical trial of the effect of postoperative intravenous fluid restriction on recovery after elective colorectal surgery. Br J Surg. 2006;93(12):1469-74.

38. Vermeulen H, Hofland J, Legemate DA, et al. Intravenous fluid restriction after major abdominal surgery: a randomized blinded clinical trial. Trials. 2009;10:50.

Section
2

Upper GI
Surgery

5
Chapter

Recent Concept in the Management of Gastric Cancer

Shameen Jaunoo

INTRODUCTION

Although the incidence of gastric cancer has steadily declined, it is frequently diagnosed at an advanced stage and globally remains the second leading cause of cancer-related death. Age-standardised mortality rates are 14.3 per 100,000 in men and 6.9 per 100,000 in women worldwide. In 2008, there were approximately 989,000 new cases of gastric cancer and 738,000 deaths worldwide.[1] The incidence shows distinct geographical variation with the highest rates in Eastern Asia (including Japan and Korea), South America and Eastern Europe and the lowest rates in North America, Western Europe and Northern and Southern Africa. Globally, it is the fourth most common cancer in men (after lung, prostate and colorectal cancer) and the fifth most common cancer in women (after breast, cervical, colorectal and lung cancer). Men are twice as likely as women to develop gastric cancer (10.9 vs 5.5 per 100,000) with a peak age incidence of 60–84 years.[2] Prognosis depends on stage at which it is detected and complete surgical resection is regarded as the only option for cure.

For tumours localised to invasion of the mucosa or submucosal at diagnosis, five-year survival rates are between 70% and 95% with exclusive surgical management. However, when extending in the gastric wall and/or there is locoregional nodal involvement, survival decreases to 20–30% at five years emphasising the fundamental importance of detecting this cancer at the earliest possible stage.[3] Technologically advanced screening programmes are needed as is improvement in the prognosis of advanced gastric cancer through multimodality treatment.

Key Points
- The incidence of gastric cancer is highest in eastern Asia, eastern Europe and South America.
- Male : Female = 2:1

CLASSIFICATION OF GASTRIC CANCER (TABLE 5.1)

Gastric cancer is a broad term encompassing multiple malignancies of varying histology and includes adenocarcinoma, lymphoma, gastrointestinal

Table 5.1: Risk factors associated with the development of gastric cancer[7-10]

Risk factor	
Helicobacter pylori	Most important modifiable risk factor (RR 2.5–3)
Smoking	RR = 1.5 Also associated with increased risk of disease recurrence
Alcohol	RR ~ 1 in light/moderate drinkers Higher with heavy intake
Dietary salt and food preservation	RR ~ 1 with each gram of salt consumed/day Salt-based preservatives and lack of refrigeration also associated with increased risk
Fruit and vegetables	Reduced intake associated with increased risk
Pernicious anaemia	RR = 6.8
Obesity	
Genetics	Hereditary diffuse gastric cancer—caused by mutation in *E-cadherin* gene. Autosomal dominant inheritance. Sixty-seven per cent cumulative risk of gastric cancer. Also increased risk of colon and lobular breast cancer. Lynch syndrome—defective DNA mismatch repair (MLH1 or MSH2 mutation). Autosomal dominant. Increased risk of gastric and colon cancer.

stromal tumours (GIST), squamous cell carcinoma, carcinoid tumours and adenocanthoma. By far the most common is adenocarcinoma, which accounts for >90% of gastric cancers and will form the focus of this review.

The Lauren system, used to histopathologically classify gastric adenocarcinoma, divides the tumour into two types: diffuse and intestinal.[4] Diffuse gastric adenocarcinoma tends to develop in younger patients, with similar incidences between men and women, and spreads by direct, lymphatic and transcoloemic routes often resulting in peritoneal disease. Submucosal infiltrative growth, a characteristic of diffuse gastric adenocarcinoma, produces a rigid, leather-bottle stomach known as linitis plastica (up to 14% of advanced gastric malignancies).[5]

Intestinal gastric adenocarcinoma tends to arise in an older population and affects men more commonly (M:F ratio 2:1). It is common in endemic regions, associated with environmental factors, atrophic gastritis and preferentially spreads haematogenously typically resulting in liver metastases. Correa et al.[6] described the multistep progression, from *Helicobacter pylori* infection and gastritis to intestinal gastric adenocarcinoma.

Macroscopically, diffuse cancers appear as ulcerating lesions endoscopically, whereas intestinal tumours tend to be exophytic, bulky lesions.

Key Point

• Adenocarcinoma is the commonest type accounting for >90% and are broadly classified as either diffuse or intestinal type.

CLINICAL MANIFESTATIONS, DIAGNOSIS AND STAGING

The vague presenting symptoms of gastric cancer account for its typically advanced stage at diagnosis. Although symptoms are generally nonspecific, patients tend to be males in the seventh to ninth decades with a history of tobacco use who report upper abdominal pain and weight loss. Dysphagia [proximal and gastro-oesophageal junction (GOJ) tumours], nausea, vomiting, haematemesis and melaena are all much less common presenting features. Rarer still are Sister Mary Joseph's nodule and Virchow's node.[11] Despite a meta-analysis[12] incorporating over 57,000 patients reporting that specific "alarm" factors had pooled sensitivities and specificities of almost 70%, their identification is likely to remain part of UK dyspepsia management guidance given their limited predictive values. As such, 2011 consensus guidelines advocate that patients ≥ 55 with new onset dyspepsia and all those with alarm features should have an urgent (within two weeks) gastroscopy.[13] A diagnosis of gastric cancer is made by visualising a mass or by histology having taken a minimum of six biopsies (Table 5.2).

Staging consists of physical examination, bloods tests and imaging. Physical examination should seek to identify skin changes or palpable masses, which invariably indicate advanced or metastatic disease. Basic blood tests include a full blood count to look for anaemia, renal biochemistry to identify electrolyte disturbances secondary to possible gastric outlet obstruction and liver function tests for possible metastases. Certain tumour markers have been shown to be poor prognosticators and indicate aggressive disease. High serum levels of markers such as carcinoembryonic antigen, CA 19-9 (carbohydrate antigen) and α-FP (alpha-fetoprotein) correlate with depth of tumour invasion, pathological stage, presence of vascular invasion and liver and lymph node metastases.[14-16]

Table 5.2: "Alarm" features suggestive of gastric cancer

New onset dyspepsia in patients >55 years of age

Family history of UGI cancer

Unintentional weight loss

Upper or lower GI bleeding

Progressive dysphagia

Iron deficiency anaemia

Persistent vomiting

Palpable mass

Palpable lymph nodes

Jaundice

A computed tomography (CT) scan of the chest, abdomen and pelvis (using oral water to ensure distension of the stomach), and intravenous contrast has a sensitivity and specificity of 74% and 99% for liver metastases, respectively, and a sensitivity of 33% for peritoneal disease (specificity 99%). The sensitivity of CT in the detection of nodal disease ranges from 50% to 95% with a specificity of 40–99%. Magnetic resonance imaging is inferior to CT for nodal staging. Positron emission tomography scanning may upstage tumours but can also be negative due to the low avidity of gastric cancers for 18F-fluoro-2-deoxyglucose and as such does not form part of the standard gastric cancer staging. It is instead reserved for oesophageal and GOJ tumours.[17]

Endoscopic ultrasound (EUS) has been shown in a meta-analysis to have a sensitivity and specificity of 86% and 91% for T staging and 69% and 84% for N staging, respectively. However, it has significant limitations for staging mucosal disease and hence does not form part of the standard staging process. It is, however, used selectively in many centres, particularly when the tumour is small and the information provided guides therapy.[18]

Finally, laparoscopy peritoneal washings for malignant cells are undertaken provided that prior imaging has indicated that the tumour is resectable. Laparoscopy is used to detect peritoneal and metastatic disease, which may have been missed on imaging, typically disease of <5 mm in diameter. Approximately 7% of gastric cancer patients will have positive cytology. A 2007 study showed that staging laparoscopy changed treatment decisions in 28% of patients after CT and EUS.[19,20]

Peritoneal cytology was incorporated into the Japanese staging system in the late 1990s following multiple studies, which showed positive cytology to be associated with disseminated disease in addition to being an independent poor prognosticator. Aside from indicating stage IV disease, positive peritoneal cytology is associated with higher T and N stages.[21-25]

Key Points

- Positive peritoneal cytology indicates disseminated and thus stage 4 disease.
- PET scanning is not routinely used in staging of gastric cancer.

TREATMENT

Multidisciplinary team (MDT) management planning is mandatory and should include surgeons, oncologists, gastroenterologists, radiologists, pathologists, nurse specialists, dieticians and a coordinator. MDT decisions should be tailored to the individual patient and must take account of patient comorbidities, nutritional status, staging investigations and patient preferences and be discussed with the patient to ensure a shared decision-making process (Table 5.3).

Table 5.3: Staging of gastric cancer

	N0	N1 (1–2)	N2 (3–6)	N3a (7–15)	N3b (≥16)	M1 (positive peritoneal cytology)
T1a (lamina propria or muscularis mucosa)	IA	IB	IIA	IIB		IV
T1b (submucosal)						
T2 (muscularis propria)	IB	IIA	IIB	IIIA		
T3 (subserosa)	IIA	IIB	IIIA	IIIB		
T4a (serosa)	IIB	IIIA	IIIB	IIIC		
T4b (adjacent organs)	IIIB		IIIC			

Source: UICC/AJCC TNM Classification, 7th edition, 2010.

Key Point
- Multidisciplinary management tailored to individual patients.

Surgery

Complete surgical resection (R0) remains the only curative modality for gastric cancer with the aim being the en-bloc removal of the primary tumour along with any direct extension and the nodal basins at risk for metastases. The UK and US guidelines recommend that all patients with regionally confined disease should undergo primary surgical resection for stage IA tumours and surgery after neoadjuvant therapy for stage II–III tumours. The extent of resection depends on preoperative staging. Cancers confined to the mucosa (T1a) are increasingly being resected endoscopically. Criteria for endoscopic resection are cancers ≤2 cm, which are histologically differentiated and not ulcerated.[26] Extensions to these criteria are being evaluated. Radical gastrectomy is required for stages 1b-3 disease. If a macroscopic proximal margin of at least 5-cm can be achieved between the GOJ and tumour, then a subtotal gastrectomy can be performed. Subtotal gastrectomy has shown identical survival and mortality results to those of total gastrectomy with a lower complication rate and fewer nutritional problems. If this is not possible, then a total gastrectomy is required. Limited resections should only be used for palliation or in the very elderly.

Key Point
- Early gastric cancer should be treated with surgery alone.

Lymphadenectomy

Controversial issues debated and studied in the last 20 years have centred upon the extent of regional lymphadenectomy (D1 vs D2). In Japan, a D2 lymphadenectomy is considered routine. The superiority of stage adjusted five-year survival rates in Japan compared to the West may be due to more extensive lymphadenectomies. Three landmark randomised prospective studies were conducted in the West to explore whether surgical technique alone, namely extent of lymphadenectomy, influenced outcome. Bonenkamp et al.[27,28] published the first randomised trial comparing D1 and D2 lymphadenectomies in Western patients (the "Dutch trial"). A total of 711 patients were randomised to receive either a D1 or D2 curative resection (380 in D1 group and 331 in D2). After a median follow-up of five years, the overall survival rates were similar between the two groups (45% vs 47% for D1 and D2, respectively, $p = .99$). However, the study showed a higher morbidity (43% vs 25%) as well as mortality (10% vs 4%) in the D2 group. In the same trial, a 15-year follow-up showed a lower rate of local recurrence and disease-related mortality in the D2 group. Factors associated with the higher morbidity in the D2 group were age over 65, male gender, type of gastrectomy and performance of a splenectomy with/without pancreatectomy. Indeed, performing a simultaneous splenopancreatectomy obscures any benefit of a D2 lymphadenectomy over a D1. A major limitation of this trial was the poor quality control of the participating surgeons with adequate expertise in performing a D2 dissection.

The British Medical Research Council ST01 was a randomised, prospective study where 737 patients were registered and underwent a staging laparotomy.[29] Of these, 400 patients were eligible and subsequently randomised to either D1 or D2 resections. The five-year overall survival rates were similar between the two groups (35% for D1 vs 33% for D2). In keeping with the Dutch trial, splenectomy and pancreatectomy were independently associated with increased morbidity and mortality.

More recently, the Italian Gastric Cancer Study Group randomised 76 patients to D1 and 86 to D2 resections with pancreas preservation.[30] They showed that complications were comparable between the two groups (10.5% for D1 vs 16.3% for D2, $p = .29$) with an overall mortality of 0.6%. This low mortality rate showed the safety and feasibility of a D2 resection with pancreatic preservation.

The sole randomised trial supporting a D3 resection was carried out by Wu et al. in Taiwan.[31] This single-centre trial randomised 221 patients to undergo either a D3 or D1 resection. Their results showed a higher morbidity in the D3 group (17.1% vs 7.3%, $p = .012$) but no significant procedure-related mortality in either group. At 5 years, overall survival was significantly better in the D3 group (59.5% vs 53.6%, $p = .041$). Although interesting, it is important to remember that when this trial was conducted, the lymph node classification system was based on nodal compartments and thus N2 and N3 nodes may have been removed in D1 resections.

In a smaller randomised trial, Robertson et al.[32] compared D1 subtotal gastrectomies to D3 total gastrectomies in 55 patients with antral cancer and found five-year survival to be better in the D1 group (45% vs 35%). Morbidity and mortality were also higher in the D3 group, which was in part attributed to complications related to pancreatectomy and splenenctomy.

Despite the negative results of the Western randomised trials, most surgeons consider a D2 advantageous because of better staging. The stage migration phenomenon, first described by Bunt et al. in 1995, was evident in the Dutch trial where up to 75% of specimens from patients in the D1 group were understaged. Thus, difference between surgical approaches not only affects survival but may also confound adjuvant therapy.

Therefore, the consensus view in the West is that a D2 lymphadenectomy should be the standard procedure, in those deemed medically fit enough, and that this should be performed in specialised centres with appropriate surgical expertise and postoperative care. Resections of the spleen and pancreas are only indicated if there is evidence of direct invasion. A splenectomy is indicated for tumours of the proximal greater curve and gastric fundus where the incidence of splenic hilar nodal involvement is likely to be high. Resection of adjacent organs is indicated where there is direct invasion or suspected transmural invasion and the patient is assessed to be fit enough for such radical surgery. Both the National Comprehensive Cancer Network and the 2011 BSG Guidelines recommend at least 15 lymph nodes be resected (Table 5.4).

Sentinel Lymph Node Biopsy (Figs. 5.1A and B)

Sentinel lymph node biopsy (SLN) is routinely used in both breast cancer and melanoma to determine whether a more formal lymph node dissection is required. Given that much of the morbidity from gastric resections relates to lymph node dissection, there has been interest in applying the principles of SLN to gastric cancer surgery. There is a significant variability in the techniques employed with the procedure being performed endoscopically or at open surgery and the injection site within the subserosa or submucosal. Dyes used include 2% patent blue, technetium-99m Sn colloid, 1% isosulfan or a combination. Detection is by direct visualisation and/or the use of a gamma probe. Data from several individual studies indicated an average of 1.5–4.1 sentinel lymph nodes being detected with sensitivities ranging from 72% to 93%, specificities of around 75%, an overall accuracy of 74–100% and a negative predictive value of 50%.[33-37] Significant limitations of sentinel lymph node biopsies in the setting of gastric cancer include a

Table 5.4: Lymph node (LN) stations

No. 1	Right paracardial LN
No. 2	Left paracardial LN
No. 3a	LN along the left gastric vessels
No. 3b	LN along the right gastric vessels
No. 4sa	LN along the short gastric vessels
No. 4sb	LN along the left gastroepiploic vessels
No. 4d	LN along the right gastroepiploic vessels
No. 5	Suprapyloric LN
No. 6	Infrapyloric LN
No. 7	LN along the left gastric artery
No. 8a	LN along the common hepatic artery (anterosuperior group)
No. 8b	LN along the common hepatic artery (posterior group)
No. 9	LN along the celiac artery
No. 10	LN at the splenic hilum
No. 11p	LN along the proximal splenic artery
No. 11d	LN along the distal splenic artery
No. 12a	LN in the hepatoduodenal ligament (along the hepatic artery)
No. 12b	LN in the hepatoduodenal ligament (along the bile duct)
No. 12p	LN in the hepatoduodenal ligament (behind the portal vain)
No. 13	LN on the posterior surface of the pancreatic head
No. 14v	LN along the superior mesenteric vein
No. 14a	LN along the superior mesenteric artery
No. 15	LN along the middle colic vessels
No. 16a1	LN in the aortic hiatus
No. 16a2	LN around the abdominal aorta (from the upper margin of the celiac trunk to the lower margin of the left renal vein)
No. 16b1	LN around the abdominal aorta (from the lower margin of the left renal vein to the upper margin of the inferior mesenteric artery)
No. 16b2	LN around the abdominal aorta (from the upper margin of the inferior mesenteric artery to the aortic bifurcation)
No. 17	LN on the anterior surface of the pancreas head
No. 18	LN along the inferior margin on the pancreas
No. 19	Infradiaphragmatic LN
No. 20	LN in the oesophageal hiatus of the diaphragm
No. 110	Paraesophageal LN in the lower thorax
No. 111	Supradiaphragmatic LN
No. 112	Posterior mediastinal LN

high false-negative rate and skip metastases. The Japan Society of Sentinel Node Navigation Surgery study group reported the findings from a multi-centre prospective trial for SLN using a dual tracer injection in 397 patients with early gastric cancer. They found a detection of 97.5%, an average of 5.6 nodes sampled, with a sensitivity of 93%, specificity, accuracy of 99% and false-negative rate of 7%.[38] The results of this trial suggest that, whilst of limited use in patients with advanced disease, patients with early gastric cancer may benefit from a limited lymphadenectomy if SLN is negative and thus a better quality of life.

Endoscopic Mucosal Resection

Endoscopic mucosal resection (EMR) is a minimally invasive method of providing curative resection whilst maintaining the gastric volume and avoiding the need for laparotomy or even laparoscopy. Postgastrectomy complications are avoided. EMR and endoscopic submucosal dissection (EDS) are indicated for patients in whom the probability of lymph node spread is low. However, there are concerns with this technique including the possibility of greater local recurrence rates and failure to obtain a staging lymphadenectomy. Furthermore, EMR often results in piecemeal resection, especially for tumours > 2 cm, and studies have found piecemeal resection to be associated with higher recurrence rates.[39,40]

Japanese treatment guidelines state that EMR is a standard treatment for differentiated mucosal gastric tumours < 2 cm and without evidence of ulceration. En bloc resection to evaluate the resection margins is required. ESD using an insulation-tipped diathermy knife (IT-knife) and the flex-knife can be used for larger tumours and thus indications for endoscopic resection may be broadened. However, it is important to remember that approximately 50% of patients in endemic countries, such as Japan and Korea, present with early gastric cancer (lesions confined to the mucosa or submucosa), whereas such presentations are rare in the West. Furthermore, early gastric cancer still carries a 10–20% risk of lymph node metastases and given this and the fact that operator experience is still low, endoscopic procedures in the West should be individualised and restricted to specialised centres with multidisciplinary input.

Laparoscopic Surgery

Laparoscopic gastrectomy remains largely investigational. A small number of randomised controlled trials have shown laparoscopic surgery to be safe with the advantage of a faster recovery. However, a meta-analysis demonstrated a reduced lymph node yield and longer operative time when compared with open surgery.[41] More studies and audits are needed as experience develops.

Robotic Surgery

Robotic-assisted surgery has been developed for use in general and paediatric surgery, gynaecology and urology. Despite having several disadvantages such as an absence of tactile feeling and cost, it does provide multi-articulated movement, reduced hand tremor, a steady camera platform and more precise dissections. In one of the largest series, Song et al.[42] reported their experience of 100 patients with early gastric cancer who underwent robot-assisted gastrectomy (33 total and 67 subtotal, with D1 lymphadenectomy) using the da Vinci system. The average operative time, length of stay and lymph node yield were 231 minutes, 7.8 days and 36.7, respectively. There were no deaths. Although other studies evaluating the safety of robotic gastrectomies have been carried out, further multi-centre, prospective and comparative trials are needed.

Adjuvant Therapy

Chemotherapy and Radiotherapy

There are limitations when advanced gastric cancer is treated solely with surgery. In the West and Asia, attempts to improve outcomes using chemotherapy and chemoradiation as neoadjuvant and adjuvant therapies have led to significant increases in survival.

The US INT-0116 trial evaluated the effectiveness of adjuvant chemoradiotherapy (CRT) after curative surgery (R0) in patients with stages IB-IV (M0) gastric and oesophagogastric junction cancer.[43] Overall survival was 36 months in the group that received both surgery and adjuvant CRT and 27 months in the group that was treated with surgery alone. Relapse-free survival was 30 months and 19 months, respectively. The results of this trial led to adjuvant CRT being accepted as the standard of care in the United States. The trial has been criticised due to the lack of surgical quality control, the low number of D2 lymphadenectomies (10%) and the high number of D0 lymphadenectomies, and thus it has been suggested that the adjuvant CRT merely compensated for suboptimal surgery.

The adjuvant chemoradiation therapy in stomach cancer (ARTIST) trial studied the effect of the addition of radiotherapy to adjuvant chemotherapy after a D2 lymphadenectomy and looked at three-year disease-free survival.[44] They found no significant difference. However, further subgroup analysis did show a survival advantage in those subjects with lymph node metastases. A further trial looking specifically at this is planned and the results eagerly awaited.

The UK MRC randomised trial (MAGIC) evaluated patients with resectable gastric, oesophagogastric junction and lower oesophageal cancers.[45] It compared surgery alone to three pre- and three post-operative cycles of epirubicin (E), cisplatin(C) and continuous intravenous 5-fluorouracil (F).

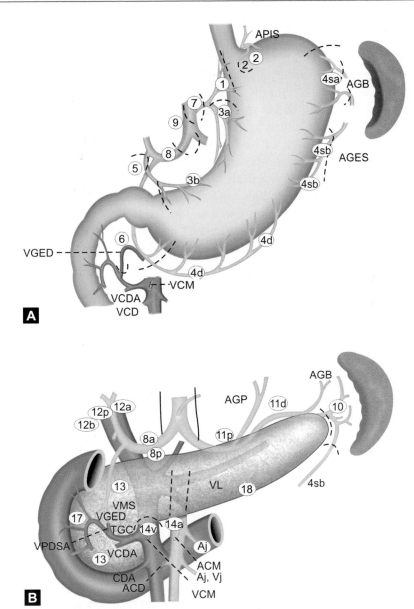

Figs. 5.1A and B: Nodal groups according to the Japanese Research Society of Gastric Cancer.

The five-year survival rate was significantly higher in the perioperative chemotherapy group (36.3%) compared with the surgery alone group (23.0%). Secondary endpoints of progression-free survival and down-staging rate were also significantly better in the chemotherapy group. Postoperative complications and 30-day mortality were similar between the two groups. A criticism of this trial is that whilst 86% of subjects completed the three courses of chemotherapy, only 42% completed postoperative ECF therapy. Results of the MAGIC trial are supported by the French phase III randomised trial (FFCD) reported in abstract form. The MAGIC trial has led to this perioperative approach being adopted as a standard of care in the United Kingdom and parts of Europe. The noninferiority of capecitabine (X) to 5-fluorouracil (F) and the advantage of not requiring an indwelling central venous catheter has resulted in many centres using an ECX regimen.

Although neoadjuvant CRT offers theoretical advantages over postoperative regimens, it remains investigational and its value has not been confirmed in randomised control trials.

The chemoradiotherapy after induction chemotherapy in cancer of the stomach (CRITICS) trial, mainly being conducted in Holland, is comparing two adjunctive therapies: perioperative ECF and adjuvant CRT.[46] The results of this study are eagerly awaited and are expected to direct adjuvant therapy in Europe and the United States.

Molecular Therapy

Molecularly targeted agents play a significant role in colorectal, breast and lung cancers. Trastuzumab, a humanised monoclonal antibody, binds selectively to the human epidermal growth factor receptor type 2 (HER2) and has improved the prognosis of HER2-positive breast cancer. HER2 overexpression has been reported in 13–20% of gastric cancers. The ToGA study examined the effectiveness of the addition of trastuzumab to chemotherapy in patients with HER2-positive gastric cancers and showed a significant difference in overall survival in the trastuzumab group compared with chemotherapy alone (13.8 months vs 11.1 months, respectively).[47] Thus, in patients with HER2 overexpression, consideration should be given to treatment with combination.

Intraperitoneal Therapy

Gastric cancer is notorious for its high recurrence rate after curative resection and for its ability to metastasise via several pathways. Recurrence following curative resection is likely due to peritoneal carcinomatosis, and certain factors have been associated with peritoneal recurrence, e.g. younger patient age, serosal involvement, diffuse type cancer and presence of infiltrative disease. Although systemic chemotherapy is the treatment of choice for disseminated disease, the blood-peritoneal barrier prevents the chemotherapeutic agents from achieving their cytotoxic effect. Intraperitoneal chemotherapy (IPC) provides the option for administering high doses of chemotherapy directly to the peritoneum whilst reducing the systemic effects. Intraperitoneal chemotherapy (IPC) can be combined with hypothermia (HIPC) and can also be administered directly after surgery (early postoperative intraperitoneal chemotherapy, EPIC). A meta-analysis of, predominantly Asian, studies on IPC, HIPC and EPIC found a significantly higher survival for HIPC compared with surgery alone, and HIPC combined with EPIC.[48] IPC was, however, associated with an increased risk of neutropaenia and intra-abdominal abscesses. In Europe, a study on gastrectomy and HIPC will shortly begin recruitment. A total of 325 patients with stage IB to IV disease with serosal involvement and ≥ 1 positive lymph node and/or positive peritoneal cytology will be randomised for three postoperative cycles of epirubicin, oxaliplatin and capecitabine (EOC) and a D2 resection, or three cycles of neoadjuvant EOC followed by a D2 gastrectomy and 30 minutes of intraperitoneal oxaliplatin.[49]

Treatment of Locally Advanced Inoperable Disease

Inoperable, locally advanced disease should be treated with palliative chemotherapy and may potentially be reassessed for surgery if a good response is achieved.

Treatment of Metastatic Disease

Patients with stage IV disease should be treated with palliative chemotherapy, which has been shown to improve survival over best supportive care alone. A meta-analysis showed the significant benefit derived by adding an anthracycline to a platinum and fluoropyrimidine doublet.[50] ECF remains amongst the most active and best-tolerated regimes. The substitution of capecitabine (X) for 5-FU (F) and oxaliplatin (O) for cisplatin (C) in the ECF regimen was evaluated in a UK National Cancer Research Institute trial and demonstrated the non-inferiority between ECF, ECX, EOF and EOX. Furthermore, the EOX combination was associated with a longer overall survival than ECF (11.2 months vs 9.9 months, respectively) and the incidence of thromboembolic phenomena was also significantly decreased by the substitution of oxaliplatin for cisplatin (7.6% vs 15.1%, $p = .0003$).[51]

In patients with recurrent disease, hypofractionated radiotherapy is effective for the palliation of bleeding, obstruction and/or pain.

It is the author's opinion that palliative gastrectomy should be limited to a small, highly selective subgroup of patients who require palliation to achieve an adequate performance status that would allow treatment with chemotherapy. It goes without saying that such decisions should be made in the context of multidisciplinary management and tailored to the individual patient.

SUMMARY

Gastric cancer remains an aggressive disease responsible for significant cancer-related mortality and, unlike the Far East, still presents at an advanced stage in the West. Surgical treatment remains the only chance of cure. Simultaneous pancreatectomy or splenectomy significantly increases morbidity and mortality and is not recommended unless there is direct organ invasion. A D2 lymphadenectomy can be performed as safely as a D1 and provides sufficient lymph nodes for staging. Perioperative chemotherapy or adjuvant chemoradiotherapy are considered a standard of care. Neoadjuvant radiotherapy or adjuvant radiotherapy alone has yet to be validated. Currently, therapies such as IPC have not gained acceptance and are still being investigated. Regardless of treatment modalities, the fundamentality of a tailored and multidisciplinary approach is unquestionable as it maximises the therapeutic options available to patients. Whilst there is still much work to be done, advances in knowledge of molecular pathways and technology will undoubtedly continue to improve patient outcomes.

Key Points

- Advanced gastric cancer is managed with perioperative chemotherapy in the United Kingdom.
- Chemotherapy and/or radiotherapy is used in palliation. Rarely should surgery be performed.

REFERENCES

1. Ferlay J, Shin HR, Bray F, et al. Estimates of worldwide burden of cancer in 2008: GLOBOCAN 2008. Int J Cancer. 2010;127:2893-917.
2. Jemal A, Bray F, Center MM, et al. Global cancer statistics. CA Cancer J Clin. 2011;61:69-90.
3. Viudez-Berral A, Miranda-Murua C, Arias-de-la-Vega F, et al. Current management of gastric cancer. Rev Esp Enferm Dig. 2012;104:134-41.
4. Lauren P. The two histological main types of gastric carcinoma: diffuse and so-called intestinal type carcinoma. ActaPatholMicrobiol Scand. 1965;64:31-49.
5. Bollschweiler E, Boettcher K, Hoelscher AH, et al. Is the prognosis for Japanese and German patients with gastric cancer really different? Cancer. 1993;71(10): 2918-25.
6. Correa P, Piazuelo MB, Carmargo MC. Etiopathogenesis of gastric cancer. Scan J Surg. 2006;95:218-24.
7. Cavaleiro-Pinto M, Peleteiro B, Lunet N, et al. Helicobacter pylori infection and gastric cardia cancer: systematic review and meta-analysis. Cancer Causes Control. 2011;22:375-87.
8. Sjodahl K, Lu Y, Milsen TI, et al. Smoking and alcohol drinking in relation to risk of gastric cancer: a population-based, prospective cohort study. Int J Cancer. 2007;120:128-32.
9. World Cancer Research Fund. Food, nutrition, physical activity, and the prevention of cancer: a global perspective. 2007. [online] Available from www. dietandcancerreport.org/cancer_resource_center/downloads/Second_Expert_ Report_full.pdf.
10. Shikata K, Kiyohara Y, Kubo M, et al. A prospective study of dietary salt intake and gastric cancer incidence in a defined Japanese population: the Hisayama study. Int J Cancer. 2006;119:196-201.

11. Anderson WF, Camargo MC, Fraumeni JF Jr, et al. Age-specific trends in incidence of noncardia gastric cancer in US adults. JAMA. 2010;303:1723-8.
12. Vakil N, Moayyedi P, Fennerty MB, et al. Limited value of alarm features in the diagnosis of upper gastrointestinal malignancy: systematic review and meta-analysis. Gastroenterology. 2006;131:390-401.
13. Allum WH, Blazeby JM, Griffin SM, et al. Guidelines for the management of oesophageal and gastric cancer. Gut. 2011;60:1449-72.
14. Mihmanli M, Dilege E, Demir U, et al. The use of tumor markers as predictors of prognosis in gastric cancer. Hepatogastroenterology. 2004;51(59):1544-7.
15. Dilege E, Mihmanli M, Demir U, et al. Prognostic value of preoperative CEA and CA 19-9 levels in resectable gastric cancer. Hepatogastroenterology. 2010;57(99-100):674-7.
16. Liu X, Cheng Y, Sheng W, et al. Clinicopathologic features and prognostic factors in alpha-fetoprotein-producing gastric cancers: analysis of 104 cases. J Surg Oncol. 2010;102(3):249-55.
17. Smyth E, Schoder H, Strong VE, et al. A prospective evaluation of the utility of 2-deoxy-2-[(18)F]fluoro-D-glucose positron emission tomography and computed tomography in staging locally advanced gastric cancer. Cancer. 2012;118:5481-8.
18. As 13
19. De Graaf GW, Ayantunde AA, Parsons SL, et al. The role of staging laparoscopy in oesophagogastric cancers. Eur J SurgOncol.2007;33:988-92.
20. Yan TD, Black D, Sugarbaker PH, et al. A systematic review and meta-analysis of the randomized controlled trials on adjuvant intraperitoneal chemotherapy for resectable gastric cancer. Ann Surg Oncol. 2007;14:2702-13.
21. Ikeguchi M, Oka A, Tsujitani S, et al. Relationship between area of serosal invasion and intraperitoneal free cancer cells in patients with gastric cancer. Anticancer Res. 1994;14(5B):2131-4.
22. Suzuki T, Ochiai T, Hayashi H, et al. Peritoneal lavage cytology findings as prognostic factor for gastric cancer. Semin Surg Oncol. 1999;17(2):103-7.
23. Burke EC, Karpeh MS Jr, Conlon KC, et al. Peritoneal lavage cytology in gastric cancer: an independent predictor of outcome. Ann Surg Oncol. 1998;5(5):411-5.
24. Hirono M, Matsuki K, Nakagami K, et al. Comparative studies on cytological and histological evaluations of disseminating peritoneal metastasis in gastric cancer. Jpn J Surg. 1981;11(5):330-6.
25. Fujimura T, Ohta T, Kitagawa H, et al. Trypsinogen expression and early detection for peritoneal dissemination in gastric cancer. J Surg Oncol. 1998;69(2):71-5.
26. Okines A, Verheij M, Allum W, et al. Gastric cancer: ESMO Clinical Practice Guidelines for diagnosis, treatment and follow-up. Ann Oncol. 2010;21(Suppl 5):v50-4.
27. Bonenkamp JJ, Hermans J, Sasako M, et al. Extended lymph-node dissection for gastric cancer.N Engl J Med. 1999; 340:908-14.
28. Bonenkamp JJ, Songun I, Hermans J, et al. Randomised comparison of morbidity after D1 and D2 dissection for gastric cancer in 996 Dutch patients. Lancet. 1995;345:745-8.
29. Cuschieri A, Weeden S, Fielding J, et al. Patients survival after D1 and D2 resections for gastric cancer: long-term results of the MRC randomised surgical trial. Surgical Co-operative Group. Br J Cancer. 1999;79(9-10):1522-30.

30. Degiuli M, Sasako M, Calgaro M, et al. Morbidity and mortality after D1 and D2 gastrectomy for cancer: interim analysis of the Italian Gastric Cancer Study Group (IGCSG) randomised surgical trial. Eur J Surg Oncol. 2004;30:303-8.
31. Wu CW, Hsiung CA, Lo SS, et al. Nodal dissection for patients with gastric cancer: a randomised controlled trial. Lancet Oncol. 2006;7(4):309-15.
32. Robertson CS, Chung SC, Woods SD, et al. A prospective randomised trial comparing R1 subtotal gastrectomy with R3 total gastrectomy for antral cancer. Ann Surg. 1994;220(2):176-82.
33. Kitagawa Y, Fujii H, Mukai M, et al. The role of the sentinel lymph node in gastrointestinal cancer. Surg Clin N Am. 2000;80(6):1799-809.
34. Orsenigo E, Tomajer V, Di Palo S, et al. Sentinel node mapping during laparoscopic distal gastrectomy for gastric cancer. Surg Endosc. 2008;22(1):118-21.
35. Hundley JC, Shen P, Shiver SA, et al. Lymphatic mapping for gastric adenocarcinoma. Am Surg. 2002;68(11):931-5.
36. Ryu KW, Lee JH, Kim HS, et al. Prediction of lymph node metastasis by sentinel node biopsy in gastric cancer. Eur J Surg Oncol. 2003;29(10):895-9.
37. Kitagawa Y, Fujii H, Kumai K, et al. Recent advances in sentinel node navigation for gastric cancer: a paradigm shift of surgical management. J Surg Oncol. 2005;90(3):147-51 [discussion: 151-2].
38. Kitagawa Y, Takeuchi H, Takagi Y, et al. Prospective multicentre trial of sentinel node mapping for gastric cancer. J Clin Oncol. 2009;27:4518.
39. Ida K, Nakazawa S, Yoshino J, et al. Multicentre collaborative prospective study of endoscopic treatment for early gastric cancer. Dig Endosc. 2004;16:295-302.
40. Ono H, Kondo H, Gotoda T, et al. Endoscopic mucosal resection for treatment of early gastric cancer. Gut. 2001;48(2):225-9.
41. Memon MA, Khan S, Yunus RM, et al. Meta-analysis of laparoscopic and open distal gastrectomy for gastric carcinoma. Surg Endosc. 2008;22:1781-9.
42. Song J, Oh SJ, Kang WH, et al. Robot-assisted gastrectomy with lymph node dissection for gastric cancer: lessons learned from an initial 100 consecutive procedures. Ann Surg. 2009;249(6):927-32.
43. Macdonald JS, Smalley SR, Benedetti J, et al. Chemoradiotherapy after surgery compared with surgery alone for adenocarcinoma of the stomach or gastroesophageal junction. N Engl J Med. 2001;345:725-30.
44. Lee J, Lim DH, Kim S, et al. Phase III trial comparing capecitabine plus cisplatin versus capecitabine plus cisplatin with concurrent capecitabine radiotherapy in completely resected gastric cancer with D2 lymph node dissection: The ARTIST trial. J Clin Oncol. 2012;30:268-73.
45. Cunningham D, Allum WH, Stenning SP, et al. Perioperative chemotherapy versus surgery alone for resectable gastroesophageal cancer. N Engl J Med. 2006;355: 11-20.
46. Dikken JL, van Sandick JW, MauritisSwellengrebel HA, et al. Neo-adjuvant chemotherapy followed by surgery and chemotherapy or by surgery and chemoradiotherapy for patients with resectable gastric cancer (CRITICS). BMC Cancer. 2011;11:329.
47. Bang YJ, van Cutsem E, Feeyereislova A, et al. Trastuzumab in combination with chemotherapy versus chemotherapy alone for treatment of HER2-positive advanced gastric or gastro-oesophageal junction cancer (ToGA): A phase 3, open label, randomised controlled trial. Lancet. 2010;376:687-97.
48. Yan TD, Black D, Sugarbaker PH, et al. A systematic review and meta-analysis of the randomised controlled trials on adjuvant intraperitoneal chemotherapy for resectable gastric cancer. Ann Surg Oncol. 2007;14:2702-13.

49. Dikken JL, Cats A, Verheiji M, et al. Randomised trials and quality assurance in gastric cancer surgery. J Surg Oncol. 2013;107:298-305.

50. Okines AF, Norman AR, McCloud P, et al. Meta-analysis of the REAL-2 and ML17032 trials: evaluating capecitabine-based combination chemotherapy and infused 5-fluorouracil-based combination chemotherapy for the treatment of advanced oesophago-gastric cancer. Ann Oncol. 2009;20:1529-34.

51. Starling N, Rao S, Cunningham D, et al. Thromboembolism in patients with advanced gastroesophageal cancer treated with anthracycline, platinum, and fluoropyrimidine combination chemotherapy: a report from the UK National Cancer Research Institute Upper Gastrointestinal Clinical Studies Group. J Clin Oncol. 2009;27:3786-93.

6
Chapter

Surgical Aspects of Gastro-oesophageal Reflux

Samrat Mukherjee, Khaled Dawas

INTRODUCTION

Gastro-oesophageal reflux disease (GORD) is caused by excessive reflux of gastric contents and sometimes biliary and pancreatic secretions into the oesophagus. A multifactorial aetiology underlies it. The importance of lifestyle factors in the aetiology of GORD has been re-emphasised in a recent systematic review.[1] It is also estimated that genetic factors contribute 18–30% to the cause of GORD.[2] Smoking, obesity and consumption of high energy rich foods have been associated with GORD.

Some degree of gastro-oesophageal reflux is normal. It manifests as physiological burping during transient relaxation of the lower oesophageal sphincter (LOS) triggered by gastric distension especially of the fundus. Small volumes of gastric contents can reflux into the postprandial oesophagus as seen on pH monitoring in asymptomatic individuals.[3] In mild to moderate GORD, structural changes at the gastro-oesophageal junction (GOJ) reduce the resistance to reflux during the transient relaxations of the LOS. In severe cases, a hiatus hernia may be present allowing large volume of gastric contents to pass unimpeded into the hiatal sac and then straining or even deep breathing may be enough to force the contents into the oesophagus.[4] Other factors that might contribute to the reflux are abnormal oesophageal motility and delayed gastric emptying.

Pathological reflux leads to typical symptoms of heartburn, upper abdominal pain and regurgitation of gastric contents into the oropharynx. However, apart from these typical symptoms, many other problems have been linked to GORD including dysphagia, hoarseness, non-cardiac chest pain, chronic cough, dental decay, pharyngitis and laryngitis. Of concern is the causal relation between oesophageal cancer and GORD via Barrett's intestinal metaplasia .The incidence of distal oesophageal adenocarcinoma is increasing.[5] Contrary to popular belief, the non-acid part of the reflux-ate has now been shown to have a role in causing oesophageal symptoms. Almost half of these patients will continue to have symptoms whilst on acid suppression treatment.[6]

INITIAL MANAGEMENT

A variety of simple measures have been proposed for management of mild symptoms. These include avoidance of precipitating factors like spicy foods, alcohol and smoking as well obesity. Although these are rarely effective for patients when they present with moderate to severe disease, they should form the first line of management.

Proton-pump inhibitors (PPIs) are much more effective in relieving symptoms and healing oesophagitis than H2 receptor antagonists (H2RA).[7,8] PPIs are associated with a greater rate of symptom relief in patients with erosive disease (70–80%) compared with patients with nonerosive reflux disease (where the symptom relief approximates 50%).[8,9]

However, patients with severe oesophagitis have a higher failure rate with these medications and many patients who do experience good relief of symptoms go on to develop "breakthrough" symptoms at a later date, eventually requiring an increase in dose. In some of these cases, bile or duodenal content reflux may play a role. Patients who respond well to PPIs may have to continue medication for life as symptoms recur quite rapidly following cessation of medications.[10] Options for GORD patients refractory to PPIs include addition of a bedtime H2RA, addition of prokinetics like metoclopramide, or a trial of baclofen.[8,11] The long-term use of PPIs has been shown to be safe and effective in spite of reports associating them to atrophic gastritis and parietal cell hyperplasia.[12-14]

Key Points

- GORD is very common and is linked to lifestyle factors.
- With most functional gastrointestinal disorders it remains important to tackle these lifestyle issues.

INVESTIGATIONS

Endoscopy

Endoscopic examination of the oesophagus is the first diagnostic investigation in patients with reflux who also have alarm symptoms. Male patients >50 years with chronic GORD and obesity have a higher than average risk of developing Barrett's oesophagus and an endoscopy is indicated.[15] An endoscopy is essential prior to anti-reflux surgery, to exclude any other pathologies.

Barium Radiographs

Radiology has important role in the investigation of motility disorders. Videofluoroscopy combined with solid and liquid bolus swallows can help in the diagnosis of pharyngeal and upper oesophageal motility disorders. It will demonstrate the presence of webs, rings, diverticula and hiatus hernias, along with the presence or absence of propagating contractions.

pH Studies

The development of miniaturised pH catheters, digital recording devices and computer analysis software has made prolonged ambulatory pH recordings widely available in clinical practice. It allows recording of acid reflux episodes as they occur and correlates patient symptom with reflux episodes.

An oesophageal pH of <4, recorded 5-cm above the LOS (defined manometrically) should be present for <5% in a 24-hour period in normal individuals.[16]

The prolonged catheter-based pH recording has its drawbacks. The catheter may interfere with eating and about 5–10% of patients are intolerant of it. Thus, the modified diet and lifestyle may not be representative of a normal day reducing reflux provoking activities.[17] The Bravo telemetry system is an endoscopically placed radiotelemetric capsule, which is better tolerated but is more expensive.

Manometry

Manometry is used to aid the placement of transnasal pH-impedance probes and is recommended before consideration of anti-reflux surgery primarily to rule out significant oesophageal dysmotility. High-resolution manometry can detect focal oesophageal dysmotility and measures the oesophagogastric pressure gradient that drives bolus transport; factors linked to improved diagnostic accuracy. The presence of weak peristaltic amplitudes or poor propagation of peristalsis is not an absolute contradiction to anti-reflux surgery. There is no evidence that a tailored approach to patient selection by, for example, choosing a partial fundoplication in patients with poor peristalsis is better.

Oesophageal Impedance Measurement

Multiple intraluminal impedance (MII) is a newer technique to detect the flow of gas and liquid through a hollow lumen. MII is often combined with pH monitoring to improve detection of pathology. Impedance-pH can be used to determine whether the refluxate is acidic, weakly acidic or weakly alkaline and can be used over a 24-hour period like pH monitoring. As it can detect non-acid reflux, MII-pH is considered the most sensitive method for reflux detection.[18] MII-pH has also been shown to improve the association of symptoms with reflux by 10–20% in GORD.[19] This helps stratify those patients who may benefit from surgical anti-reflux treatment.[20]

Measurement of Duodenogastric Reflux

Although acid reflux is responsible for the bulk of oesophageal symptoms, symptoms can occur without acid being detected in the refluxate. The measurement of bile reflux with the Bilitec 2000 recorder (Synectics, Stockholm, Sweden) is similar to an ambulatory pH recording. It uses spectrophotometry to detect the absorbance of bilirubin as an indirect measure of bile reflux. Studies have shown that bile reflux is only responsible for a minority (7%) of symptoms.[21]

SURGICAL MANAGEMENT

Who to Operate on?

Patient selection for anti-reflux surgery is the key to ensuring a good surgical outcome. All patients who undergo anti-reflux surgery should have evidence of reflux demonstrated on pH studies. Patients with reflux symptoms and negative pH studies should be carefully counselled before embarking on surgery.[22]

The GORD patients who wish to discontinue medical therapy may be referred for surgery. There are those with large hiatus hernias, reflux with respiratory complications and Barrett's oesophagus with reflux who may also be considered.[23]

The best surgical responses are seen in patients with typical symptoms that demonstrate good response to PPI therapy, have abnormal pH studies with good symptom correlation.[24] In this group, long-term remission rates can be expected to be comparable and in some cases statistically superior to medical therapy. In a long-term follow-up of a randomised controlled trial comparing medical to surgical therapy for GORD, 92% of the patients in the medical arm were on medical therapy compared with 62% of the surgical cohort at 10 years.[25] In a 12-year follow-up of patients randomised to fundoplication versus omeprazole, 53% of the surgery cohort were in remission compared with 45% of the medically treated patients ($p = .02$), although symptoms of gas-bloat syndrome remained more common in the surgical cohort.[26] The result of a number of trials comparing laparoscopic anti-reflux surgery with medical treatment suggests better symptom control in the surgery group.[27,28] In a Cochrane review, four randomized trials with over 1,200 subjects randomized to medical or surgical therapy were included. All reported significant improvements in GORD-specific quality of life parameters after surgery although data were not combined.[29]

Key Points

- Careful patient workup before offering surgery is vital.
- All patients should have thorough oesophageal physiology studies.

Surgical Procedures

The principle of surgical management is the creation of a mechanical anti-reflux barrier between the oesophagus and the stomach. It entails mobilising the lower oesophagus and wrapping the fundus of the stomach, either partially or wholly, around the oesophagus and narrowing the hiatus.

Nissen Fundoplication

This is the most commonly performed anti-reflux procedure worldwide. The original operation entailed mobilisation of the oesophagus from the diaphragmatic hiatus, reduction of any hiatus hernia, preservation of the vagus and mobilisation of the posterior gastric fundus behind the oesophagus without dividing the short gastric vessels and performing a complete 360° wrap of 5-cm length. Most surgeons now agree that a fundoplication of 1–2 cm in length achieves an optimal outcome. This is in conjunction with a posterior crural repair, which still allows for oesophageal dilatation during swallowing.[30]

Posterior Partial Fundoplication

A variety of partial fundoplications have been described in an attempt to minimise the risk of dysphagia and gas-bloat. Toupet described a 270° posterior fundoplication where the edges of the fundus are sutured to the left and right lateral wall of the oesophagus, as well as to the right diaphragmatic pillar. Lind described a similar procedure with a 300° posterior fundoplication.

Anterior Partial Fundoplication

Several anterior fundoplications have been described, with the purpose of reducing the incidence of dysphagia and other side effects. Some are historic and rarely performed nowadays (Belsey Mark IV procedure). The Dor procedure is an anterior fundoplication (180°), which is performed with a cardiomyotomy for achalasia.

Surgical Controversies

The relative merits of complete versus partial fundoplication have been debated for many years. On one hand, some argue that the "total" Nissen procedure has a higher incidence of dysphagia and gas-bloat, but on the other hand, it is a more effective anti-reflux procedure. Lundell et al. reported that dysphagia rates and reflux control at five-year follow-up for a Nissen and posterior partial fundoplication were similar, although re-operation was more common after Nissen fundoplication. The results were similar even at 11-year follow-up.[31] Zornig reported a trial of total versus partial fundoplication on patients with normal and abnormal oesophageal motility. A good outcome was obtained in about 90% of patients and short-term dysphagia was more common after total fundoplications, with no correlation between preoperative oesophageal motility and outcome.[32,33] This is likely to be where the dysmotility is secondary to reflux. Studies comparing Nissen with anterior partial fundoplication have shown similar results.[34]

Further controversy focused on the need to divide the short gastric vessels. There is no strong evidence that dividing the short gastric vessels leads to better functional outcomes. In fact, division of the vessels produced a poorer outcome due to gas-bloat related events in a single randomised trial.[35]

Key Points

- The choice of type of fundoplication remains a personal preference.
- Patients should be counselled carefully about the risks of gas bloat and dysphagia preoperatively.
- The decision to divided the short gastric vessels is often made at the time of surgery.

Outcomes After Surgery

The results of several large series with long-term follow-up have confirmed that laparoscopic Nissen fundoplication is effective, and at 10 years still achieves an excellent clinical outcome in >85–90% of patients. Laparoscopic surgery reduces pain and shortens the recovery period after surgery.[36,37]

One of the most common side effects of a fundoplication is gas-bloat (15–20%). A recent meta-analysis concluded that the prevalence of postoperative dysphagia and inability to belch were significantly lower in patients undergoing partial fundoplication compared with patients undergoing a total fundoplication.[38] Because fundoplication produces a one-way valve, patients are usually warned about not being able to belch effectively and so need to be cautious about drinking fizzy drinks. Similarly, they may not be able to vomit. Consequently, these patients experience an increased passage of flatus.[39]

Complications

Paraoesophageal hiatus herniation is reported in the early postoperative period following laparoscopic anti-reflux surgery in up to 7% of cases.[40] Extended oesophageal dissection into the mediastinum during laparoscopic procedures, increased risk of breaching the left pleural membrane and less postoperative pain are factors, which have been implicated in allowing the stomach to slide into the left hemithorax during coughing, vomiting or any exertion in the early postoperative period (Figs. 6.1A and B). Routine hiatal

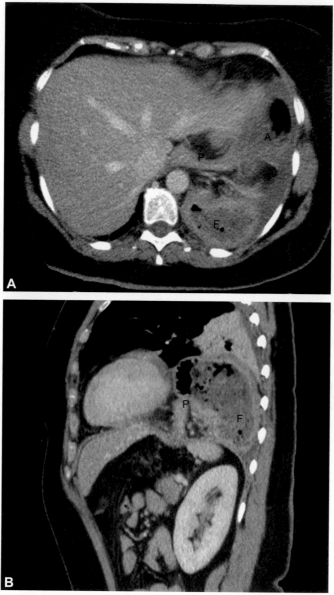

Figs. 6.1A and B: (A) Computed tomographic scan showing migration of the whole stomach up into the mediastinum following a fundoplication; (B) Sagittal section showing the migrated stomach above the diaphragm. (P: Pylorus; A: Antrum; F: Fundus).

repair has been shown to reduce the incidence by almost 80% and excessive strain on the repair should be avoided in the early postoperative period by the use of antiemetics and avoiding heavy lifting/straining.[40]

Severe early dysphagia requiring surgical revision occurs and conversion from a Nissen to a partial fundoplication or, in extremes, undoing the fundoplication may be required. A tight "wrap" may be seen on a contrast swallow study (Fig. 6.3). More common is a tight diaphragmatic hiatus either due to a tight crural repair, which requires a laparoscopic release of one or more crural sutures, or due to scarring requiring endoscopic dilatation or laparoscopic division of the hiatal ring.[41]

An intra-operative pneumothorax may occur in up to 2% of patients from injury during the retro-oesophageal dissection. This is more common with large hiatus hernias and may occasionally need a tube thoracostomy.

Injury to the vagus nerve may be responsible for postoperative diarrhoea and symptoms of delayed gastric emptying. Iatrogenic oesophageal and gastric perforation complicate around 1% of cases in most series. Rarer complications, such as, vascular or liver injury, pulmonary embolism and bilobed stomach have all been described.[30]

Key Points

- Early paraoesophageal herniation is a rare but problematic complication.
- Most patients will experience dysphagia postoperatively.
- Significant dysphagia two months postoperatively requires careful investigation.

Failure of Anti-Reflux Surgery

It is difficult to get an accurate estimate of the rates of redo anti-reflux surgery as most studies are of small volume or from a single centre. Lafullarde published a reoperation rate of >10% in patients who underwent a fundoplication between 1991 and 1994.[42] More recently, reoperation rates of approximately 5% have been reported.[43-45]

The main reason for failed anti-reflux procedures is inadequate patient selection. Other causes of a poor outcome include failure to recognise delayed gastric emptying; failure to recognise a short oesophagus or wide hiatus; failure to recognise oesophageal dysmotility/endstage reflux disease and failure in the technical aspects of the procedure.

Common surgical pitfalls include:
- The fundus being wrapped around the stomach instead of the oesophagus
- Incomplete oesophageal mobilisation to obtain a 2–3 cm of abdominal oesophagus
- Incomplete mobilisation of the gastric fundus (some cases may necessitate division of the short gastric vessels) resulting in a tight fundoplication
- Incomplete crural closure or tight crural stitches leading to strangulation of the crural muscles (use of pledgets and meshes is advocated by some).

Horgan et al. described a classification system: Type I failures occur with displacement of the GOJ through the oesophageal hiatus with (type IA) or without (type IB) the wrap. Type II failures are defined as failure secondary to a para-oesophageal hernia. Type III failures occur as a result of malposition of the wrap at the time of the initial surgery, usually on the cardia of the stomach.[46]

Fundoplication failures not included in this classification system also include wraps that are too tight or loose, or failures secondary to unrecognized oesophageal or gastric dysmotility.[47]

Key Points

- Surgical failure is linked to poor patient selection.
- Technical faults in fashioning the fundoplication should also be considered.

Management of Recurrent or Persistent Symptoms After Surgery

Patients present with persistent symptoms, recurrent symptoms or new symptoms. Persistent symptoms are common in patients with atypical symptoms of GORD. Failure to relieve preoperative symptoms is likely due to an initial misdiagnosis. Recurrence of symptoms following an initial relief after surgery suggests the possibility of a disrupted, slipped or herniated fundoplication. New-onset symptoms, like persistent dysphagia, are linked to a tight, misplaced or twisted wrap.

To clarify the aetiology an upper gastrointestinal barium study (video fluoroscopy) and endoscopy is essential (Figs. 6.2 and 6.3). It is often necessary to repeat the 24-hour oesophageal pH study as well. Oesophageal high definition manometry can help in the diagnosis of a slipped fundoplication.

Laparoscopic revisional surgery is technically challenging. Operative times, length of hospital stay and morbidity is greater in revisional surgery compared to the primary procedure. Outcomes of revisional surgery are not as good as the primary procedure with an increased incidence of gas bloat and dysphagia and poorer control of symptoms.[47]

Mediastinal oesophageal mobilisation is essential in patients with a shortened oesophagus and sometimes a Collis gastroplasty is required to get an adequate length of abdominal oesophagus. A gastropexy to anchor the fundoplication to the crura is occasionally used to minimise the risk of wrap migration. The use of pledget reinforcement to the crural or gastric sutures can help avoid early disruption of the repair.

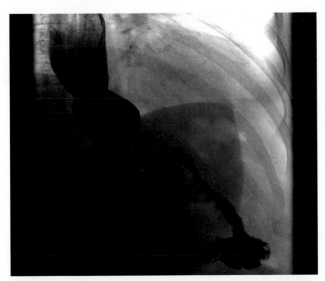

Fig. 6.2: Barium swallow showing distal oesophageal holdup proximal to a smooth stricture in the region of the wrap. This suggests a very tight fundoplication wrap.

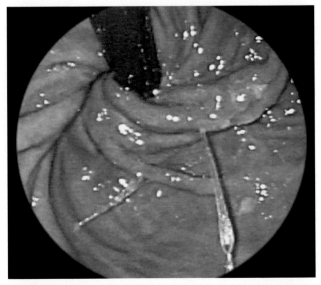

Fig. 6.3: Normal endoscopic appearance of a Nissen fundoplication.

Key Points

- Revisional surgery is very challenging.
- Revisional surgery should be preceded by repeating most UGI investigations.
- Clinical outcomes after revisional surgery are less satisfactory.

ENDOSCOPIC PROCEDURES

There have been a few attempts at endoscopic therapies. Procedures which narrow the GOJ have disappointing clinical outcomes and more recent endoscopic (transoral) partial fundoplication techniques are being described with more promise.

Radio Frequency

The Stretta procedure used a device to apply radiofrequency energy to the GOJ to cauterise the oesophageal muscle and cause fibrosis, thereby aiming to tighten the GOJ. Subsequent randomized trial of the Stretta and sham endoscopy showed no difference at six-month follow-up.[48]

Endoscopic Suturing

The EndoCinch procedure entails the endoscopic placement of two 3-mm-deep sutures into the gastric mucosal folds immediately below the GOJ, to create pleats to narrow the region. However, studies showed that reflux was cured in only a minority of patients. In a randomized sham controlled trial, symptom scores improved following the EndoCinch procedure, but the results did not compare well with the outcomes of laparoscopic anti-reflux surgery.[49]

The NDO Plicator uses a flexible overtube, which can be retroflexed in the stomach. A screw penetrates and retracts the GOJ and full thickness plication of the cardia is done to narrow the GOJ. This is secured with a special suture. A sham controlled trial actually showed a significant reduction in oesophageal acid exposure from 10% to 7% at three months, but the degree of improvement was inferior to a surgical anti-reflux procedure.[50]

Endoscopic Fundoplication

EsophyX: The EsophyX procedure aims to construct a fundoplication. An endoscope is passed through the device and both are passed transorally into the stomach. The endoscope is retroflexed and a screw anchors tissue at the GOJ for caudal retraction. A plastic arm then compresses the fundus against the oesophagus and multiple polypropylene fasteners are passed between the oesophagus and the fundus to anchor them together. Fasteners are applied starting from the greater curvature and advancing radially towards the lesser curvature to produce a 200–300° anterior partial fundoplication.

Clinical experience with this device is limited to a few centres in Europe. Limited published clinical studies suggest that in some patients a fundoplication can be constructed. However, the short-term results are still inferior to a laparoscopic fundoplication.[51]

Medigus: The Medigus SRS procedure is another endoscopic construction of an anterior partial fundoplication. It uses a purpose built disposable endoscope that contains stapling and ultrasound devices. The tip can retroflex more acutely than a standard gastroscope, allowing it to meet the side of the instrument. The end of the device can be locked to the side, forming two halves of a stapler and ultrasound is used to measure the gap between the tip and the side, to allow optimum staple placement. The fundus of the stomach is stapled to the side of the oesophagus, 2–3 cm above the GOJ.[52]

NEWER PROCEDURES

LINX Reflux System

The LINX device consists of a series of titanium beads with magnetic cores sealed inside. The beads are linked by titanium wires to form a flexible and expandable ring with a "Roman arch" configuration. Each bead can move independently of the other, creating a dynamic implant that mimics the physiological movements of the GOJ without limiting its range of motion. The attractive force between closed beads is approximately 40g and decreases exponentially with distance. It is available in different sizes and is can reach almost twice its diameter when all beads are separated.

For reflux to occur, the intragastric pressure must overcome both LOS pressure and the magnetic bonds of the device, creating a resistance to opening. This device, whilst augmenting the LOS, allows expansion to accommodate a food bolus or the escape of elevated gastric pressure seen with belching or vomiting. This provides control of reflux without compromising the physiologic function of the LES.[53]

The LINX device is implanted laparoscopically under general anaesthesia. It is placed in a tunnel between the posterior vagus and the oesophageal wall and the opposing ends are then brought to the anterior surface of the oesophagus and connected together. It may be performed as a day case.

Sphincter augmentation using the LINX Reflux has shown efficacy up to 4 years in the reduction of the amount of pathologic oesophageal acid exposure in a small number of subjects. This device has been approved by the Food and Drug Administration, USA based on a clinical study in 100 GORD patients. This study found that performance of LINX resulted in consistent symptom relief and pH control with markedly fewer side effects than traditional laparoscopic fundoplication in well-selected patients.[54]

EndoStim LES Stimulation System

In selected patients with GORD, electrical stimulation of the LOS results in raised LOS pressure without interfering with the LOS relaxation. The stimulation electrodes are placed in the LOS and a pulse generator is implanted laparoscopically. LOS stimulation is delivered in 6–12, 30-min sessions each day. Initial reports suggest that it reduces oesophageal acid exposure and good symptom control at 12-month follow-up.[55]

REFERENCES

1. Dent J, El-Serag HB, Wallander MA, et al. Epidemiology of gastro-oesophageal reflux disease: a systematic review. Gut. 2005;54(5):710-7.
2. Fox M, Forgacs I. Gastro-oesophageal reflux disease. BMJ. 2006;332(7533):88-93.
3. Demeester TR, Johnson LF, Joseph GJ, et al. Patterns of gastroesophageal reflux in health and disease. Ann Surg. 1976;184(4):459-70.
4. Sifrim D. Relevance of volume and proximal extent of reflux in gastro-oesophageal reflux disease. Gut. 2005;54:175-8.
5. Lagergren J, Bergstrom R, Lindgren A, et al. Symptomatic gastroesophageal reflux as a risk factor for esophageal adenocarcinoma. N Engl J Med. 1999;340:825-31.
6. Sifrim D. Acid, weakly acidic and non-acid gastro-oesophageal reflux: differences, prevalence and clinical relevance. Eur J Gastroenterol Hepatol. 2004;16(9):823-30.
7. North of England Dyspepsia Guideline Development Group. Dyspepsia: management of dyspepsia in adults in primary care. London: National Institute for Health and Clinical Excellence; 2004.
8. Katz PO, Gerson LB, Vela MF. Guidelines for the diagnosis and management of gastroesophageal reflux disease. Am J Gastroenterol. 2013;108(3):308-28.
9. Gralnek IM, Dulai GS, Fennerty MB, et al. Esomeprazole versus other proton pump inhibitors in erosive esophagitis: a meta-analysis of randomized clinical trials. Clin Gastroenterol Hepatol. 2006;4:1452-8.
10. Schindlbeck NE, Klauser AG, Berghammer G, et al. Three year follow up of patients with gastrooesophageal reflux disease. Gut. 1992;33:1016-9.
11. Orr WC, Goodrich S, Wright S, et al. The effect of baclofen on nocturnal gastroesophageal reflux and measures of sleep quality: a randomized, cross-over trial. Neurogastroenterol Motil. 2012;24:553-9.
12. Klinkenberg-Knol EC, Nelis F, Dent J, et al. Long-term omeprazole treatment in resistant gastroesophageal reflux disease: efficacy, safety, and influence on gastric mucosa. Gastroenterology. 2000;118:661-9.
13. van Grieken NC, Meijer GA, Weiss MM, et al. Quantitative assessment of gastric corpus atrophy in subjects using omeprazole: a randomized follow-up study. Am J Gastroenterol. 2001;96(10):2882-6.
14. Cats A, Schenk BE, Bloemena E, et al. Parietal cell protrusions and fundic gland cysts during omeprazole maintenance treatment. Hum Pathol. 2000;31(6):684-90.
15. Becher A, Dent J. Systematic review: ageing and gastro-oesophageal reflux disease symptoms, oesophageal function and reflux oesophagitis. Aliment Pharmacol Ther. 2011;33:442-54.
16. Bodger K, Trudgill N. Guidelines for oesophageal manometry and pH monitoring. BSG Guidelines Gastroenterol. 2006;1-11.
17. Wong WM, Bautista J, Dekel R, et al. Feasibility and tolerability oftransnasal/per-oral placement of the wireless pH capsule vs traditional 24h oesophageal pH monitoring—a randomized trial. Aliment Pharmacol Ther. 2005;21(2):155-63.
18. Shay S, Richter J. Direct comparison of impedance, manometry, and pH probe in detecting reflux before and after a meal. Dig Dis Sci. 2005;50(9):1584-90.
19. Bredenoord AJ, Weusten BL, Curvers WL, et al. Determinants of perception of heartburn and regurgitation. Gut. 2006;55(3):313-18.
20. MainieI, Tutuian R, Agrawal A, et al. Combined multichannel intraluminal impedance-pH monitoring to select patients with persistent gastro-oesophageal reflux for laparoscopic Nissen fundoplication. Br J Surg. 2006;93(12):1483-7.

21. Koek GH, Tack J, Sifrim D, et al. The role of acid and duodenal gastroesophageal reflux in symptomatic GERD. Am J Gastroenterol. 2001;96(7):2033-40.
22. Waring JP, Hunter JG, Oddsdottir M, et al. The preoperative evaluation of patients considered for laparoscopic antireflux surgery. Am J Gastroenterol. 1995;90:35-8.
23. Gurski RR, Peters JH, Hagen JA, et al. Barrett's esophagus can and does regress after antireflux surgery: a study of prevalence and predictive features. J Am Coll Surg. 2003;196:706-12.
24. Oelschlager BK, Quiroga E, Parra JD, et al. Long-term outcomes after laparoscopic antireflux surgery. Am J Gastroenterol. 2008;103:280-7.
25. Spechler SJ, Lee E, Ahnen D, et al. Long-term outcome of medical and surgical therapies for gastroesophageal reflux disease: follow-up of a randomized controlled trial. JAMA 2001;285:2331-8.
26. Lundell L, Miettinen P, Myrvold HE, et al. Comparison of outcomes twelve years after antireflux surgery or omeprazole maintenance therapy for reflux esophagitis. Clin Gastroenterol Hepatol. 2009;7:1292-8.
27. Mahon D, Rhodes M, Decadt B, et al. Randomized clinical trial of laparoscopic Nissen fundoplication compared with proton-pump inhibitors for treatment of chronic gastro-oesophageal reflux. Br J Surg. 2005;92:695-9.
28. Mehta D, Bennett J, Mahon D, et al. Prospective trial of laparoscopic Nissen fundoplication versus proton pump inhibitor therapy for gastroesophageal reflux disease: seven year follow-up. J Gastrointest Surg. 2006;10:1312-6.
29. Wileman SM, McCann S, Grant AM, et al. Medical versus surgical management for gastro-oesophageal reflux disease (GORD) in adults. Cochrane Database Syst Rev. 2010;CD003243.
30. Engström Cl, Cai W, Irvine T, et al. Twenty years of experience with laparoscopic antireflux surgery. Br J Surg. 2012;99(10):1415-21.
31. Lundell L, Abrahamsson H, Ruth M, et al. Long term results of a prospective randomized comparison of total fundic wrap (Nissen-Rosetti) or semifundoplication (Toupet) for gastro-oesophageal reflux. Br J Surg. 1996;83:830-5.
32. Zornig C, Strate U, Fibbe C, et al. Nissen versus Toupet laparoscopic fundoplication. Surg Endosc. 2007;21:1985-90.
33. Strate U, Emmermann A, Fibbe C, et al. Laparoscopic fundoplication: Nissen versus Toupet two-year outcome of a prospective randomized study of 200 patients regarding preoperative oesophageal motility. Surg Endosc. 2007;22:21-30.
34. Ludemann R, Watson DI, Game PA, et al. Laparoscopic total versus anterior 180 degree fundoplication—five year follow-up of a prospective randomized trial. Br J Surg. 2005;92:240-3.
35. Yang H, Watson DI, Lally CJ, et al. randomized trial of division versus non-division of the short gastric vessels during laparoscopic Nissen fundoplication—10 year outcomes. Ann Surg. 2008;247:38-42.
36. Kelly J, Watson DI, Chin K, et al. Laparoscopic Nissen fundoplication—clinical outcomes at 10 years. J Am Coll Surg. 2007;205:570-5.
37. Cowgill SM, Gillman R, Kraemer E, et al. Ten year follow up after laparoscopic Nissen fundoplication for gastroesophageal reflux disease. Am Surg. 2007;73:748-52.
38. Ramos RF, Lustosa SA, Almeida CA, et al. Surgical treatment of gastroesophageal reflux disease: total or partial fundoplication? Systematic review and meta-analysis. Arq Gastroenterol. 2011;48:252-60.
39. Gotley DC, Smithers BM, Rhodes M, et al. Laparoscopic Nissen fundoplication—200 consecutive cases. Gut. 1996;38:487-91.

40. Watson DI, Jamieson GG, Devitt PG, et al. Paraoesophageal hiatus hernia: an important complication of laparoscopic Nissen fundoplication.Br J Surg. 1995;82:521-3.
41. Wetscher GJ, Glaser K, Wieschemeyer T, et al. Tailored antireflux surgery for gastroesophageal reflux disease: effectiveness and risk of post-operative dysphagia. World J Surg. 1997;21:605-10.
42. Lafullarde T, Watson DI, Jamieson GG, et al. Laparoscopic Nissen fundoplication: five-year results and beyond. Arch Surg. 2001;136(2):180-4.
43. Byrne JP, Smithers BM, Nathanson LK, et al. Symptomatic and functional outcome after laparoscopic reoperation for failed antireflux surgery. Br J Surg. 2005;92(8):996-1001.
44. Dutta S, Bamehriz F, Boghossian T, et al. Outcome of laparoscopic redo fundoplication. Surg Endosc. 2004; 18(3):440-3.
45. Funch-Jensen P, Bendixen A, Iversen MG, et al. Complications and frequency of redo antireflux surgery in Denmark: a nationwide study, 1997–2005. Surg Endosc. 2008;22(3):627-30.
46. Horgan S, Pohl D, Bogetti D, et al. Failed anti-reflux surgery: what have we learnt reoperations? Arch Surg. 1999;134:809-17.
47. Hatch KF, Daily MF, Christensen BJ, et al. Failed fundoplications. Am J Surg. 2004;188:786-91.
48. Corley DA, Katz P, Wo JM, et al. Improvement of gastroesophageal reflux symptoms after radiofrequency energy: a randomized sham controlled trial. Gastroenterology. 2003;125:668-76.
49. Schwartz MP, Wellink H, Gooszen HG, et al. Endoscopic gastroplication for the treatment of gastro-oesophageal reflux disease: a randomized, sham-controlled trial. Gut. 2007;56:20-8.
50. Rothstein R, Filipi C, Caca K, et al. Endoscopic full thickness plication for the treatment of gastroesophageal reflux disease: a randomized, sham-controlled trial. Gastroenterology. 2006;131:704-12.
51. Cadiere GB, Rajan A, Germay O, et al. Endoluminal fundoplication by a transoral device for the treatment of GERD: a feasibility study. Surg Endosc. 2008;22(2):333-42.
52. http://www.medigus.com/healthcare-professional
53. Ganz R, Peters J, Horgan S, Bemelman W, Dunst C, Edmundowicz S, et al. Esophageal sphincter device for gastroesophageal reflux disease. N Engl J Med. 2013;368:719-27.
54. Lipham JC, Demeester TR, Ganz RA, et al. The LINX reflux management system: confirmed safety and efficacy now at 4 years. Surg Endosc. 2012;26:2944-9.
55. Rodríguez L1, Rodriguez P, Gómez B, et al. Long-term results of electrical stimulation of the lower esophageal sphincter for the treatment of gastroesophageal reflux disease. Endoscopy. 2013;45(8):595-604.

7
Chapter

Determining Resectability in Pancreatic Cancer

Giles Bond-Smith, Giuseppe Kito Fusai

INTRODUCTION

Pancreatic cancer is the 10th most common cancer in the United Kingdom and the 13th most common cancer worldwide. However, it is the fifth most common cause of cancer-related mortality in the East and the fourth most common cause of cancer-related mortality in the West.[1-3] Over 8,000 new cases of pancreatic cancer are diagnosed every year in the United Kingdom. The incidence rate is currently 9.7 per 100,000 in the United Kingdom, with its peak between the seventh and eight decades and is rare under the age of 40. With a slight bias to younger men and older women, the male to female ratio is 1:1.[4,5]

Surgical resection remains the only hope of cure for patients diagnosed with pancreatic cancer. It has an overall survival of 0.4%[6] to 4%,[7] with those patients amenable to surgical resection and adjuvant chemotherapy having a five-year survival of up to 23%, as reported by the ESPAC1 study.[8] As pancreatic cancer often presents late, <20% of patients have surgically resectable disease at the time of diagnosis.[4] Of the inoperable ones, approximately two thirds present with distant metastases and the remaining one third with locally advanced disease.[9] In one study involving 799 newly diagnosed patients only 18% were considered suitable for curative resection, whereas no five-year survivors were recorded in the inoperable group.[10] Defining resectability is therefore one of the most important and crucial aspects in the management of pancreatic cancer.

DEFINITIONS

Historically localised pancreatic tumours have been classified as either resectable or unresectable. It is primarily the relationship of the pancreatic cancer to the vessels that defines resectability. Over the last two decades the terms "locally advanced" and "borderline resectable" pancreatic cancer have come in to use.

To help fully understand what these terms mean it is important to be familiar with the TNM staging system, which is listed below.

Table 7.1: The American joint committee on cancer stage groupings and TNM definitions.		
Stage	*TNM*	*Description*
0	Tis, N0, M0	Tis = Carcinoma in situ
IA	T1, N0, M0	T1 = Tumour limited to the pancreas, ≤2 cm in greatest dimension
IB	T2, N0, M0	T2 = Tumour limited to the pancreas, >2 cm in greatest dimension
IIA	T3, N0, M0	T3 = Tumour extends beyond the pancreas but without involvement of the coeliac axis or superior mesenteric artery
IIB	T1, N1, M0 T2, N1, M0 T3, N1, M0	N1 = Regional lymph node metastasis
III	T4, any N, M0	T4 = Tumour involves the coeliac axis or the superior mesenteric artery (unresectable primary tumour)
IV	any T, any N, M1	M1 = Distant metastasis

Locally advanced pancreatic cancer is described as having left the boundaries of the pancreas and invaded locally adjacent structures such as major blood vessels, lymph nodes, bowel or the bile duct, without evidence of distant metastatic disease. Involvement of locoregional lymph nodes is not regarded as a surgical contraindication, whereas if the para-aortic or other distant lymph nodes are affected, these should be regarded as metastases. Locally advanced pancreatic cancer may or may not be resectable and would include T3 and T4, of the above TNM classification, whereas T1 and T2 are considered resectable tumours.

In 2001, Mehta et al. reported a study in which patients were classified as "marginally resectable" based on radiographic evidence of partial portal vein (PV), superior mesenteric vein (SMV) or mesenteric arterial involvement.[11] These radiographic findings were felt to make surgery technically challenging to gain a resection margin free of tumour. This study became one of the first descriptions of "borderline resectable" disease.

Since then two subtly different definitions have become established in the current literature. In 2006, the MD Anderson Cancer Center (MDACC) group reported their definition of borderline resectable tumours.[12] Two years later, the American HepatoPancreatoBiliary Association (AHPBA)/ Society of Surgical Oncology (SSO)/Society for Surgery of the Alimentary Tract (SSAT) Groups published a Consensus document.[13] Both the MDACC and the AHPBA/SSO/SSAT groups defined borderline resectable pancreatic cancers on the basis of a limited radiographic interface between the tumour and the superior mesenteric artery (SMA) (Fig. 7.1) or hepatic artery (HA). The definitions from the two groups however differ on the extent of venous involvement required to classify borderline tumours, as the MDACC group describes any venous involvement as resectable disease and only occlusion

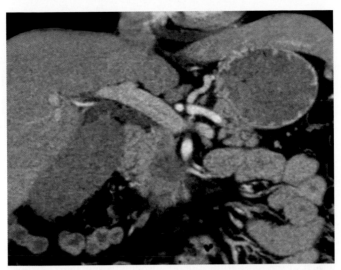

Fig. 7.1: Coronal computed tomography (CT) demonstrates involvement of the lateral wall of the superior mesenteric artery (SMA) for approximately 180°. Patient was considered "borderline resectable" and is currently having neo-adjuvant chemoradiotherapy.

of the SMV or PV (with the possibility of reconstruction) as borderline.[14] These two sets of criteria to define borderline disease have ultimately been incorporated into the National Comprehensive Cancer Network (NCCN) Guidelines for pancreatic cancer treatment.

The current NCCN Criteria for resectability of pancreatic cancer are listed below and describe the differences between resectable, borderline resectable and unresectable pancreatic cancer.[15] Recently, these criteria have also been supported and recommended by the International Study Group for Pancreatic Surgery.[16]

Resectable

- *Arterial*: Clear fat planes around the coeliac axis (CA), SMA and HA.
- *Venous*: The SMV or PV abutment but no distortion of the vessels.

Borderline Resectable

- *Arterial (Head of Pancreas)*: Gastroduodenal artery encasement up to the HA with either short segment encasement or direct abutment of the HA but without extension to the CA. Tumour abutment of the SMA <180° of the circumference of the vessel wall.
- *Arterial (Body/Tail of Pancreas)*: Less than 180° involvement of the circumference of the CA.
- *Venous*: Venous involvement of the SMV or PV with distortion or narrowing of the vein or occlusion of the vein with suitable vessel proximal and distal, allowing for safe resection and replacement (Fig. 7.2).

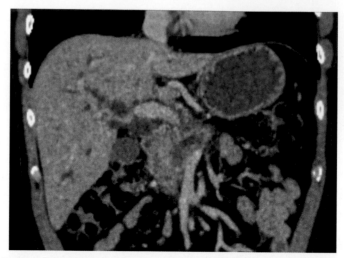

Fig. 7.2: Coronal CT demonstrating superior mesenteric vein (SMV) involvement, with short segment of occlusion of the portomesenteric vein. Biliary dilatation is noticed as the tumour is obstructing the distal bile duct.

Unresectable

- *Arterial (Head of Pancreas)*: Greater than 180° encasement of the circumference of the SMA or any CA abutment.
- *Arterial (Body/Tail of Pancreas)*: SMA or CA encasement >180°.
- *Arterial (Any Part of the Pancreas)*: Aortic invasion or encasement.
- *Venous*: Unreconstructable SMV and/or PV.
- *Nodal Status*: Metastases to lymph nodes beyond the field of resection should be considered unresectable.

The ambiguity of terms such as "abut" or "encase", used within both the MDACC and AHPBA/SSO/SSAT classification systems as well as in the NCCN guidelines, has caused some difficulty in standardising radiological reports.[12,14] To simplify and standardise the language to describe borderline resectable pancreatic cancer, the Alliance for Clinical Trials in Oncology/Southwest Oncology Group/Eastern Cooperative Oncology Group and the Radiation Therapy Oncology Group have recently proposed an alternative definition. This definition is currently being used in a pilot study of border-line resectable pancreatic cancer (Alliance Trial A021101).

According to this definition borderline resectable pancreatic cancer must meet one or more of the following:[12]

1. An interface exists between tumour and the SMV or PV measuring ≥180° of the vessels wall circumference, and/or reconstructable venous occlusion.
2. An interface exists between tumour and the SMA measuring <180° of the vessel wall circumference.

3. A reconstructable, short-segment interface of any degree exists between tumour and the common HA.
4. An interface exists between tumour and the coeliac trunk measuring < 180° of the vessel wall circumference.

In summary, borderline resectability is determined by minimal arterial, and up to, more extensive venous involvement, which might preclude a potentially curative resection. Resectional surgery should aim to achieve complete tumour clearance (R0), although several studies have shown that the resection margin status is not the most important prognostic indicator, with patients undergoing R0 and R1 resections having a similar survival.[17-20]

The role of neo-adjuvant oncological treatment in patients with borderline pancreatic cancer is still not defined, with different studies suggesting a survival benefit and higher R0 rates with preoperative chemotherapy, radiotherapy or a sequential combination of both.[11,21-24] In 2013, Takahashi et al. highlighted the potential benefit of neo-adjuvant chemoradiotherapy in borderline resectable pancreatic cancer. They reported 54% of patients in the borderline resectable group were resected post neo-adjuvant chemotherapy with a 98% R0 resection rate. This produced a 34% five-year survival rate in this group.[25]

An international RCT, the ESPAC-5 trial (ISRCTN89500674), is currently recruiting patients with borderline resectable pancreatic cancer, randomised to surgery versus neo-adjuvant oncological treatment followed by surgery.

- TNM Classification used for staging pancreatic adenocarcinoma.
- Borderline resectability based on interface between tumour and vascular structures.
- Different criteria have been suggested to define borderline resectable disease but NCCN guidelines most frequently used.

INCREASING RESECTABILITY RATES

Survival for pancreatic cancer has not changed in the last 40 years. However, with advancement in surgical technique and improvement in perioperative care surgical mortality has reduced to <5%. In high volume, specialised centres, postoperative mortality rates of 2–3% have been reported.[26] To try and increase resectability and improve the long-term survival for patients with pancreatic cancer, extensive surgical procedures have been developed, mainly involving vascular reconstruction techniques. The journey to this point has not been straightforward or without complication.

Birkmeyer et al.[26] first reported aggressive surgery for borderline resectable pancreatic cancer with the first SMV resection and reconstruction in 1951. Asada et al. followed this by performing a radical pancreaticoduodenectomy (PD) and PV resection in 1963.[27] In 1973, Fortner first described the regional pancreatectomy. This involved a total pancreatectomy, radical lymph node clearance, combined PV resection (type 1) and/or combined arterial resection and reconstruction (type 2).[28]

Due to the higher morbidity and mortality associated with these technically demanding and complex operations, and with no discernable benefit in survival, the West temporarily abandoned this aggressive surgical practice. More recently, however, to improve resectability rates of pancreatic cancer, there has been growing interest in revisiting these procedures by experienced teams, in high volume centres and in selected cohorts of patients.

Venous Resection

Venous involvement by pancreatic cancer is not considered a contraindication to surgical resection. In 2004, Yekebas et al.[29] demonstrated a perioperative mortality and long-term survival similar to those reported in patients undergoing conventional surgery with no PV resection.

However, a pancreatic resection requiring venous reconstruction is technically challenging and may be associated with a higher morbidity. Despite the evidence from Tseng et al. there was concern amongst surgeons as to the feasibility of the procedure.

These concerns were tackled by Zhou et al. in 2008[30] and Siriwardana and Siriwardena et al.,[31] with a meta-analysis in 2012, when they reported that there was no statistically significant difference in intraoperative blood loss and transfusion requirement between patients undergoing pancreatic resection with and without PV reconstruction.[29,30]

In support of this Ravikumar et al. have recently published a large UK multicentre retrospective cohort study comparing, PD with venous resection (PDVR) and surgical bypass for T3 adenocarcinoma of the head of the pancreas. Morbidity was similar between the PDVR and PD groups, with only delayed gastric emptying and patients requiring blood transfusion being greater in the PDVR group.[9]

With the technical and safety aspects of these procedures placed to one side, outcomes needed to be addressed.

In 2006, Siriwardana reported a large systematic review of 1646 patients who had undergone portal-SMV resection during pancreatectomy for cancer. They concluded that, with the high rate of nodal metastases and the low five-year survival rates, once the PV is involved cure is unlikely even with radical surgery.[31] This paper may be criticised as many of the series had only a few cases reported, the review covered a long historical period when surgical technique was different and most importantly approximately 15% of the series included patients with simultaneous venous and arterial resections.

The implication of this systematic review is one of surgical futility if there is venous involvement. Reports have disputed this view as patients with stage III pancreatic cancer have a median survival time of 10–12 months, shorter than the median survival reported in many series of PV resection for pancreatic cancer.[9,17,32] Indeed, to date, several studies have shown that PV resection in patients with pancreatic cancer has comparable survival to standard pancreatectomy and is a safe procedure when performed in specialist HPB Units. Most importantly, it confers a survival advantage over surgical palliation, as demonstrated also by two randomised controlled trials.

In the first one, Lygidakis et al. compared en bloc splenopancreatic and venous resection versus palliative gastrobiliary bypass and reported two-year survival rates of 81.8% and 0%, respectively,[33] whereas the randomised controlled trial by Doi et al. in 2008 was closed early when interim analysis showed a clear survival benefit for PDVR with chemoradiotherapy compared with chemoradiotherapy with or without a surgical bypass.[34]

This led an expert consensus statement to conclude that PDVR and reconstruction is the standard of practice for pancreatic adenocarcinoma locally involving the PV/SMV, providing that adequate inflow and outflow veins are present, the tumour does not involve the SMA or HA and an R0/R1 resection is reasonably expected (Figs. 7.3A and B).[35,36]

Arterial Resection

Since the original description from Fortner in 1973 several authors have published their experience of arterial resection in borderline resectable pancreatic cancer.

In 2007, Hirano et al. reported their long-term follow-up for patients undergoing distal pancreatectomy with en bloc CA resection (DP-CAR) (Figs. 7.4A and B). They reported one-year and five-year survival rates of 71% and 42%, respectively, and concluded that DP-CAR offers a high R0 resectability rate and may potentially achieve complete local control in selected patients.[37]

Bachellier et al., in 2011, matched a group of patients undergoing pancreatectomy with arterial resection to conventional pancreatectomy and demonstrated similar three-year survival rates.[38] Also in 2011, Bockhorn et al. reported one of the largest series on pancreatectomy with simultaneous arterial resection ($n = 29$) and concluded that there was no overall difference in disease-specific survival for patients who underwent arterial reconstruction versus those patients who underwent pancreatectomy alone. Also both resection groups had better survival than the non-resected patients who underwent a palliative bypass.[39] Despite these positive reports, to date there is not sufficient evidence to suggest arterial resection as a standard of care in patients with borderline disease.

Mollberg et al. also, in 2011, summarised the experience of pancreatectomy with arterial resection in a systematic review and meta-analysis.

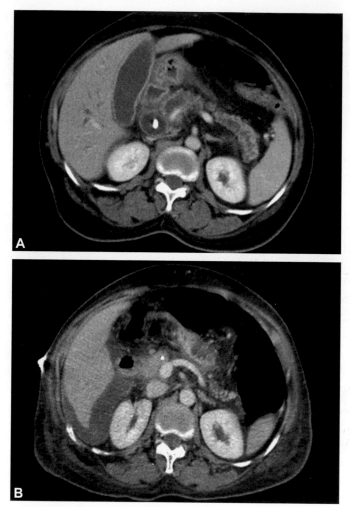

Figs. 7.3A and B: (A) Axial section showing extensive involvement of portomesenteric vein with bile duct stenting. (B) Whipples procedure has been performed with reconstruction of the portal vein, using an interposition graft from the internal jugular, and re-implantation of the splenic vein.

This report included 26 studies, a total of 2609 patients, with considerable heterogeneity between them. Three hundred and sixty-six, out of the 2609 patients underwent an arterial resection and reconstruction in conjunction with a pancreatectomy.

The results of the review suggested a significantly increased perioperative morbidity and a mortality rate compared with the one observed in patients undergoing standard pancreatectomy. A subgroup analysis confirmed this risk when arterial resection was compared with the PV reconstruction.

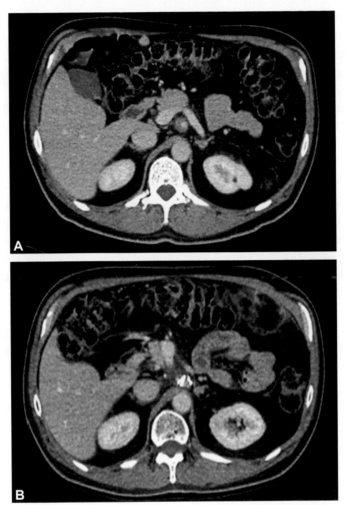

Figs. 7.4A and B: Axial computed tomography (CT) demonstrating soft tissue around the coeliac axis (A). Patient underwent a distal pancreatectomy with en-bloc coeliac artery resection after sequential neo-adjuvant chemotherapy and chemora-diation (B).

Significantly poorer survival outcomes at one year (49.1%), three years (8.3%) and five years (0%) were also demonstrated in this study. However, a potential medium term survival benefit was suggested when comparing pancreatectomy with arterial resection to medical palliation.[35]

The study by Mollberg et al. is a detailed analysis of the available data from 1973 to 2010. The conclusion is that for tumours involving the arterial structures, including the SMA and the common HA, arterial resection may be justified in highly selected patients, preferably in the context of studies involving neo-adjuvant protocols of chemo and radiotherapy. A prospective registry to allow accurate analysis of outcome data for patients undergoing a pancreatectomy with arterial resection was also proposed. This is currently being developed and is part of a multicentred prospective study.[40]

- Resectability rate can be increased by extending surgical indications, particularly in patients with borderline disease.
- Portomesenteric venous reconstruction should be the standard of care.
- Arterial resection still controversial and appropriate only within prospective studies in highly selected patients.

CONCLUSIONS

Although borderline pancreatic cancer currently encompasses both arterial and venous involvement, the two types of vascular reconstruction have completely different risks and outcomes.

The first is widely accepted as a standard of care in patients with radiological abutment or even encasement if a surgical option to reconstruct the vessel exists. The second, on the other hand, is highly controversial with very few centres performing this type of surgery. Newly designed prospective studies integrated with medical oncological treatments will hopefully provide an answer in the near future as to whether arterial resection should be performed in patients with pancreatic cancer.

REFERENCES

1. Gurusamy KS, Kumar S, Davidson BR, et al. Resection versus other treatments for locally advanced pancreatic cancer. Cochrane Database Syst Rev. 2014;2:Cd010244.
2. Parkin DM, Bray FI, Devesa SS. Cancer burden in the year 2000. The global picture. Eur J Cancer. 2001;37 Suppl 8:S4-66.
3. Parkin DM, Bray F, Ferlay J, et al. Global cancer statistics, 2002. CA Cancer J Clin. 2005;55(2):74-108.
4. Coupland VH, Kocher HM, Berry DP, et al. Incidence and survival for hepatic, pancreatic and billiary cancers in England between 1998 and 2007. Cancer epidemiology. 2012;36(4):e207-14.
5. Bond-Smith G, Banga N, Hammond TM, et al. Pancreatic adenocarcinoma. BMJ (Clinical research ed). 2012;344:e2476.
6. Bramhall SR, Allum WH, Jones AG, et al. Treatment and survival in 13,560 patients with pancreatic cancer, and incidence of the disease, in the West Midlands: an epidemiological study. Br J Surg. 1995;82(1):111-5.
7. Jemal A, Murray T, Samuels A, et al. Cancer statistics, 2003. CA Cancer J Clin. 2003;53(1):5-26.
8. Ryu JK, Hong SM, Karikari CA, et al. Aberrant MicroRNA-155 expression is an early event in the multistep progression of pancreatic adenocarcinoma. Pancreatology. 2010;10(1):66-73.
9. Ravikumar R, Sabin C, Abu Hilal M, et al. Portal vein resection in borderline resectable pancreatic cancer: a United Kingdom multicenter study. J Am Coll Surg. 2014;218(3):401-11.

10. Geer RJ, Brennan MF. Prognostic indicators for survival after resection of pancreatic adenocarcinoma. Am J Surg. 1993;165(1):68-72; discussion -3.
11. Mehta VK, Fisher G, Ford JA, et al. Preoperative chemoradiation for marginally resectable adenocarcinoma of the pancreas. J Gastrointest Surg. 2001;5(1): 27-35.
12. Katz MH, Marsh R, Herman JM, et al. Borderline resectable pancreatic cancer: need for standardization and methods for optimal clinical trial design. Ann Surg Oncol. 2013;20(8):2787-95.
13. Callery MP, Chang KJ, Fishman EK, et al. Pretreatment assessment of resectable and borderline resectable pancreatic cancer: expert consensus statement. Ann Surg Oncol. 2009;16(7):1727-33.
14. Cooper AB, Tzeng CW, Katz MH. Treatment of borderline resectable pancreatic cancer. Current treatment options in oncology. 2013;14(3):293-310.
15. Tempero MA, Malafa MP, Behrman SW, et al. Pancreatic adenocarcinoma, version 2.2014. Journal of the National Comprehensive Cancer Network : JNCCN. 2014;12(8):1083-93.
16. Bockhorn M, Uzunoglu FG, Adham M, et al. Borderline resectable pancreatic cancer: a consensus statement by the International Study Group of Pancreatic Surgery (ISGPS). Surgery. 2014;155(6):977-88.
17. Raut CP, Tseng JF, Sun CC, et al. Impact of resection status on pattern of failure and survival after pancreaticoduodenectomy for pancreatic adenocarcinoma. Ann Surg. 2007;246(1):52-60.
18. Fusai G, Warnaar N, Sabin CA, et al. Outcome of R1 resection in patients undergoing pancreatico-duodenectomy for pancreatic cancer. Eur J Surg Oncol. 2008;34(12):1309-15.
19. Neoptolemos JP, Stocken DD, Dunn JA, et al. Influence of resection margins on survival for patients with pancreatic cancer treated by adjuvant chemoradiation and/or chemotherapy in the ESPAC-1 randomized controlled trial. Ann Surg. 2001;234:758-68.
20. Jarufe NP, Coldham C, Mayer AD, et al. Favourable prognostic factors in a large UK experience of adenocarcinoma of the head of the pancreas and periampullary region. Dig Surg. 2004;21:202-9.
21. Auriemma WS, Berger AC, Bar-Ad V, et al. Locally advanced pancreatic cancer. Seminars in oncology. 2012;39(4):e9-22.
22. Warshaw AL, Fernandez-del Castillo C. Pancreatic carcinoma. N Engl J Med. 1992;326(7):455-65.
23. Small W Jr., Berlin J, Freedman GM, et al. Full-dose gemcitabine with concurrent radiation therapy in patients with nonmetastatic pancreatic cancer: a multicenter phase II trial. J Clin Oncol. 2008;26(6):942-7.
24. Stokes JB, Nolan NJ, Stelow EB, et al. Preoperative capecitabine and concurrent radiation for borderline resectable pancreatic cancer. Ann Surg Oncol. 2011;18(3):619-27.
25. Takahashi H, Ohigashi H, Gotoh K, et al. Preoperative gemcitabine-based chemoradiation therapy for resectable and borderline resectable pancreatic cancer. Ann Surg. 2013;258(6):1040-50.
26. Birkmeyer JD, Finlayson SR, Tosteson AN, et al. Effect of hospital volume on in-hospital mortality with pancreaticoduodenectomy. Surgery. 1999;125(3): 250-6.
27. Asada S, Itaya H, Nakamura K, et al. Radical pancreatoduodenectomy and portal vein resection. Report of two successful cases with transplantation of portal vein. Arch Surg. 1963;87:609-13.

28. Fortner JG. Regional resection of cancer of the pancreas: a new surgical approach. Surgery. 1973;73(2):307-20.
29. Yekebas EF, Bogoevski D, Cataldegirmen G, et al. En bloc vascular resection for locally advanced pancreatic malignancies infiltrating major blood vessels: perioperative outcome and long-term survival in 136 patients. Ann Surg. 2008;247(2):300-9.
30. Zhou Y, Zhang Z, Liu Y, et al. Pancreatectomy combined with superior mesenteric vein-portal vein resection for pancreatic cancer: a meta-analysis. World J Surg. 2012;36(4):884-91.
31. Siriwardana HP, Siriwardena AK. Systematic review of outcome of synchronous portal-superior mesenteric vein resection during pancreatectomy for cancer. Br J Surg. 2006;93(6):662-73.
32. Tseng JF, Raut CP, Lee JE, et al. Pancreaticoduodenectomy with vascular resection: margin status and survival duration. J Gastrointest Surg. 2004;8(8):935-49; discussion 49-50.
33. Lygidakis NJ, Singh G, Bardaxoglou E, et al. Mono-bloc total spleno-pancreaticoduodenectomy for pancreatic head carcinoma with portal-mesenteric venous invasion. A prospective randomized study. Hepatogastroenterology. 2004;51(56):427-33.
34. Doi R, Imamura M, Hosotani R, et al. Surgery versus radiochemotherapy for resectable locally invasive pancreatic cancer: final results of a randomized multi-institutional trial. Surg Today. 2008;38(11):1021-8.
35. Evans DB, Farnell MB, Lillemoe KD, et al. Surgical treatment of resectable and borderline resectable pancreas cancer: expert consensus statement. Ann Surg Oncol. 2009;16(7):1736-44.
36. Christians KK, Lal A, Pappas S, et al. Portal vein resection. Surg Clin North Am. 2010;90(2):309-22.
37. Hirano S, Kondo S, Hara T, et al. Distal pancreatectomy with en bloc celiac axis resection for locally advanced pancreatic body cancer: long-term results. Ann Surg. 2007;246(1):46-51.
38. Bachellier P, Rosso E, Lucescu I, et al. Is the need for an arterial resection a contraindication to pancreatic resection for locally advanced pancreatic adenocarcinoma? A case-matched controlled study. J Surg Oncol. 2011;103(1):75-84.
39. Bockhorn M, Burdelski C, Bogoevski D, et al. Arterial en bloc resection for pancreatic carcinoma. Br J Surg. 2011;98(1):86-92.
40. Mollberg N, Rahbari NN, Koch M, et al. Arterial resection during pancreatectomy for pancreatic cancer: a systematic review and meta-analysis. Ann Surg. 2011;254(6):882-93.

Section 3

Lower GI Surgery

8
Chapter

Enhanced Recovery Following Colorectal Resection

Vimal Hariharan, Daren Francis

INTRODUCTION

Laparoscopic colorectal surgery has led the way to the establishment of the enhanced recovery programme (ERP) or "fast track" pathway as it is sometimes known. Indeed, its demonstrated success in colorectal surgery has allowed it to be adopted into a wide range of allied surgical specialities.

From its conception in early 2000, Kehlet coined the phrase "ERP" and published his remarkable findings reducing operative morbidity and reducing length of stay to a minimum.[1] The combination of the ERP and laparoscopic surgery are synergistic and to this day the vast majorities of colorectal units in the United Kingdom follow an abbreviated form of the original ERP.

What Is the ERP?

Traditional hospital stay of 10–14 days for major bowel resection had been accepted as the normal practice until fairly recently. However, in 2000, Basse and Kehlet[3] described a clinical pathway to accelerate recovery after colonic resection, which dramatically cut down length of stay. Their study described a median stay of two days with a readmission rate of 15%.

After study and development a consensus on what the ERP core protocol contained was formed by Fearon et al. in 2005.[2]

The principles of care are based on:
1. Preoperative interventions
2. Perioperative interventions
3. Postoperative care.

Enhanced recovery following colorectal surgery aims to minimise the stress response on the body and return gut function as rapidly as possible. It can be thought of as a combination of elements, which together reduce the morbidity and length-of-stay postcolorectal resection. Many of the interventions aim to address postoperative ileus, which is a major hurdle to overcome for recovery following colorectal surgery. In addition to minimising the stress response to surgery the aim is to speed recovery and return

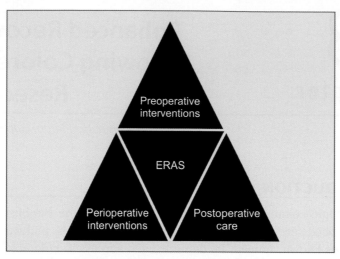

Fig. 8.1: Principles of ERAS.

to normal function, thus minimising complications and improving overall outcomes. Over the last decade there has been an increasing consensus as to what denotes an ERP. It is important to stress that a multidisciplinary approach is mandatory for enhanced recovery after surgery (ERAS) to function. This must incorporate willingness from hospital staff as well as the patient and the relatives. A relatively recent role is that of the "Enhanced Recovery Nurse Specialist". They are central and coordinate the multi-modal aspects of care including input from allied specialities such as the wards nurses, pain team, dieticians and physiotherapists.

Preoperative Interventions

Major surgery produces a stress on the body, which leads to increased metabolic demand and nitrogen consumption. Typically, the patient will be in a catabolic state for the first few days postoperatively and will lose lean muscle mass rapidly as the body tries to replenish its nitrogen stores.

The introduction of "carbohydrate loading" two hours preoperatively decreases postoperative insulin resistance and negative nitrogen balance, thus reducing postoperative complications. Several randomised trials have shown this benefit along with the importance of maintaining postoperative oral nutrition as well.[4]

Patients find bowel preparation difficult to tolerate and troublesome to manage. Along with the dehydration and potential renal sequelae of the mass osmotic loss of fluids, patients themselves find the discomfort and disturbance the night prior to their surgery impacts on their physical and emotional status. It stands to reason that "a good night's sleep" before major surgery should be sought if at all possible. Multiple systematic reviews and meta-analyses have assessed the role of bowel preparation and concluded that mechanical bowel prep does not reduce anastomotic leakage and may increase wound infection rates.[5]

Most surgeons now use bowel preparation for patients undergoing anterior resection and total mesorectal excision (as a column of faeces between the stoma and defunctioned anastomosis could theoretically increase the chance of anastomotic dehiscence). For left sided or high rectal anastomoses a simple enema at the time of surgery is employed.

Key Points

Preoperative care incorporates optimisation of the patient, ensuring adequate hydration and minimisation of starvation.
- Admission on the day of surgery.
- Judicious use of bowel preparation.
- Carbohydrate pre-loading.
- Careful counselling of the patient.

Perioperative Care

Perioperative care starts with minimising the insult of surgery. With the advent and progress of laparoscopic surgery, wounds are now much smaller, access to parts of the abdomen that previously would have needed larger incisions can be accomplished with incisions that do not need closing. There is less tissue manipulation, retraction and stress.[6] This facilitates reduced anaesthetic and analgesic requirements. This in turn leads to reduced bed rest and an earlier return to normal function.

The laparoscopic approach is only a facet of the ethos of enhanced recovery. Certainly, it lends itself to the programme but in no way does an operation not performed laparoscopically (wholly or partly) exclude itself from using the tools of enhanced recovery. As discussed earlier enhanced recovery is making its way into all the surgical specialities and is not confined to colorectal resection solely.

The perioperative preparation starts in the anaesthetic room. The anaesthetist plans the anaesthetic in close conjunction with the surgeon. Consideration is given as to the type of agents used; pre-medication is now avoided; agents with long half-lives and opiates are minimised. The patient is minimally starved and is relatively well hydrated. Perioperative analgesia is planned; mid-thoracic epidural or transversus abdominus plane blocks and patient controlled analgesia (PCA) are selected depending on the unit's preference. There are issues however with epidural anaesthesia. Hübner et al. randomised 128 patients to Epidural vs PCA and found the epidural arm to slow down recovery and increase the need for vasopressor support.[8] Patient pain scores on day one were unchanged. Combined with the accepted 10% failure rate of epidurals they concluded that this mode of anaesthesia should not be recommended. Total intravenous anaesthesia is becoming more commonplace, and agents such as remifentanil have ultra-short half-lives of 4 minutes leading to a "fast on, fast off" effect. Other methodologies exist such as single shot spinal anaesthesia, infusion catheters and peripheral antagonists, but the principle remains the same, i.e. one should aim for a comfortable patient postoperatively who is able to return to function rapidly.

Nasogastric drainage and postoperative drains should be avoided if possible. This aids early patient mobillisation. No benefit for routine anastomotic drainage has been found by a recent Cochrane review.[7] Intra-operative use of noninvasive monitoring should be used for goal directed fluid replacement. Central venous and arterial line catheters are no longer standard for the American Society of Anaesthesiologists grade I and II patients.

Fluid balance is a topic of much controversy with many contradictory findings from trials. However, the evidence is clear that gut function and tissue healing, morbidity and hospital stay are adversely affected by the overuse on intravenous fluid therapy.[9] This along with Brandstrup's[10] work shows a clear survival benefit in those patients who are fluid restricted as opposed to those that receive large sodium and volume loads. It was shown that a patient who received < 2 L and 77 mmol of sodium per day had improved gastric emptying and reduced complications. It is not clear as to the cause of this effect, but we must remember that during surgical stress the body retains salt and water via anti-diuretic hormone and renin–angiontensin–aldosterone pathways. Goal directed fluid therapy intra-operatively optimises cardiac output and improves outcome.[11] Use of trans-oesophageal Doppler allows for the measurement of stroke volume and cardiac output. Its use has been validated to give accurate changes in cardiac output as opposed to an absolute true value. Fluid therapy can then be directed at keeping pre-load optimised (and hence Starling's curve within its maximal contractility) to reduce the work of the myocardium. It is now routine to administer relatively small amounts of colloid frequently whilst guided by the oesophageal Doppler readings. An important point to note is that postoperative hypotension should never be blamed on the epidural anaesthesia, a surgical cause should be excluded in the first instance. Although commonplace, hypotension due to epidurals is caused by the blocking of sympathetic fibres in the epidural space. This causes dilation of peripheral blood vessels and decreased peripheral vascular resistance. If longstanding hypotension is problematic then vasopressors are a better compensator then large volumes of fluid. Decreasing the epidural rate to allow the patient to feel pain is never a solution.

Surgical technique is evolving to produce minimal trauma to the patient. Often though a surgeon's desire for minimising the scar or extraction site can lead to overcomplicating the operation itself. Therefore, a balance needs to be met with minimally invasive surgery including the total operating time, number of ports, extraction site size, benefit to the patient, etc. Specimen extraction should be accomplished by the smallest incision possible such as transverse incision for colonic resections and either a modified Pfannenstiel or lower midline for rectal resections. Infra-umbilical incisions are preferable as they cause less postoperative pain.

Key Points
- Tailor the type of anaesthesia to the patient and operation.
- Avoid long-acting opiates.
- Laparoscopic surgery reduces the overall stress response.
- Goal directed fluid therapy reduces complications.

Postoperative Interventions

As described adequate pain relief is essential. The patient must be motivated and pain free to do the things we ask of them. A well-sited epidural, minimal tissue handling, small surgical scars and no "tubes" to tie the patient down are all beneficial. Early mobilisation with the patient sitting out of bed the following postoperative day is desirable. An established care plan with motivated staff who can guide and encourage the patient provides the best care. We find the establishment of colorectal nurse specialists who visit the patient daily and monitor progress invaluable.

Early feeding is a cornerstone of ERAS and discontinuation of IV fluids should be done as soon as feasible. Commencement of carbohydrate drinks should supplement normal dietary intake. The patient should be monitored for early postoperative complications and rapid intervention offered.

Patients should be monitored for the development of an ileus, and if identified oral feeding should be curtailed and supportive measures put in place such as IV fluid replacement with high concentrations of electrolytes along with nasogastric drainage. Discharge planning should commence as early as possible. After discharge telephone follow-up at 24 hours is arranged with the Nurse Specialist. This gives the patient confidence that they are still under an umbrella of care. Patients also have ease of access to the surgical team via the ERAS Nurse Specialist and can have close follow-up and rapid assessment if not progressing along the expected path.

SPECIAL CONSIDERATIONS

Many surgeons apply ERAS selectively and proportionally. Whilst this is not incorrect and we feel a proportionate response is merited as one can sometimes predict, which patient will tolerate the protocol and which will not. This comes with experience but we feel that elements of ERAS can be beneficial to all patient groups.

Application of ERAS in the elderly has been hitherto thought of as unwise. Bagnall et al.[12] performed a systematic review, which included the findings of 16 studies. They found ERAS to be safe in the elderly population (>65) with ERAS promoting a reduction in complications and shortened length of stay.

Many of the randomised controlled trials that have looked into the efficacy of ERAS are critical of the readmission rate. However, a recent systematic review by Nicholson et al.[13] looked at over 5,000 patients. They concluded that there was a reduction in the length of stay, a reduction in the 30-day complication rate but no difference in all cause mortality, major complications or readmission rate.

Enhanced recovery following colorectal resection has delivered a framework with which patient centred care can flourish. It divides the patient journey into stages and ensures the surgical stress inflicted onto the patient is minimised. However, one should remember that although all of the interventions are recommendations to the patient, and have been proven to shorten stay, minimise risk and reduce morbidity, a tailored approach with the patient's abilities and wishes should be employed.

REFERENCES

1. Nygren J, Hausel J, Kehlet H, et al. A comparison in five European Centres of case mix, clinical management and outcomes following either conventional or fast-track perioperative care in colorectal surgery. Clin Nutr. 2005;24(3):455-61.
2. Fearon KC, Ljungqvist O, Von Meyenfeldt M, et al. Enhanced recovery after surgery: a consensus review of clinical care for patients undergoing colonic resection. Clin Nutr. 2005;24(3):466-77.
3. Basse L, HjortJakobsen D, Billesbolle P, et al. A clinical pathway to accelerate recovery after colonic resection. Ann Surg. 2000;232(1):51-7.
4. Svanfeldt M, Thorell A, Hausel J, et al. Randomised clinical trial of the effect of preoperative oral carbohydrate treatment on postoperative whole-body protein and glucose kinetics. Br J Surg. 2007;94(11):1342-50.
5. Guenaga KF, Matos D, Castro AA, et al. Mechanical bowel preparation for elective colorectal surgery. Cochrane Database Syst Rev. 2005;(1):CD001544.
6. Veenhof AA, Vlug MS, van der Pas MH, et al.: Surgical stress response and postoperative immune function after laparoscopy or open surgery with fast track or standard perioperative care: a randomised trial. Ann Surg. 2012;255(2):216-21.
7. Jesus EC, Karliczek A, Matos D, et al. Prophylactic anastomotic drainage for colorectal surgery. Cochrane Database Syst Rev. 2004;(4):CD002100.
8. Hübner M, Blanc C, Roulin D, et al. Randomized clinical trial on epidural versus patient-controlled analgesia for laparoscopic colorectal surgery within an enhanced recovery pathway [published online ahead of print Aug 12, 2014]. Ann Surg. PMID: 25119117.

9. Lobo DN, Bostock KA, Neal KR, et al. Effect of salt and water balance on recovery of gastrointestinal function after elective colonic resection: a randomised controlled trial. Lancet. 2002;359(9320):1812-8.

10. Brandstrup B, Tonnesen H, Beier-Holgersen R, et al. Effects of intravenous fluid restriction on postoperative complications: comparison of two perioperative fluid regimens: a randomised assessor-blinded multicenter trial. Ann Surg. 2003;238(5):641-8.

11. Walsh SR, Tang T, Bass S, et al. Doppler-guided intra-operative fluid management during major abdominal surgery: systematic review and meta-analysis. Int J Clin Pract. 2008;62(3):466-70.

12. Bagnall NM1, Malietzis G, Kennedy RH, et al. A systematic review of enhanced recovery care after colorectal surgery in elderly patients [published online ahead of print July 18, 2014]. Colorectal Dis. doi: 10. 1111/codi.12718.

13. Nicholson A, Lowe MC, Parker J, et al. Systematic review and meta-analysis of enhanced recovery programmes in surgical patients. Br J Surg. 2014;101(3): 172-88.

9

Chapter

Management of Fistula-in-ano

Clarisa Choh, Claire Warden, Thomas Dudding

INTRODUCTION

Despite being one of the oldest reported medical conditions, the management and treatment of anal fistula is still evolving. The prevalence of the disease is unclear as the majority of epidemiological studies cite incidence within poorly defined populations. There are well-documented links between fistula-in-ano and Crohn's disease; however, the majority of fistulae seen in clinical practice are cryptoglandular in origin. Whilst cryptoglandular fistulae are perceived to be easier to manage, they can still be a challenge to treat; the management of this type of fistula will be the focus of this chapter. Anal fistulae caused by carcinoma, tuberculosis, HIV and other infections are rare, but they do need to be considered in unusual or persistent disease.

PATHOGENESIS

Fistula are believed to be infective in origin, although recent evidence suggests that there is a paucity of bacteria found within fistula tracts and chronic bacterial infection may not be the pathological process that leads to maintenance of the disease.[1] Despite this, the cryptoglandular theory, based on the studies performed by Tucker, Hellwig and Eisenhammer is still central in our understanding of the how fistulae are initially formed. It is believed that anal sepsis originates from cystic dilatation of anal intramuscular glands due to blockage of draining ducts. This leads to formation of an intersphincteric abscess that then tracks in the direction of the longitudinal anal muscle as its fibres penetrate into the internal and external anal sphincter muscles. Around 40% of patients presenting with an acute perianal abscess will develop a chronic fistula after incision and drainage.[2]

DIAGNOSIS

Initial management of fistula-in-ano involves establishing the diagnosis, delineating the anatomy and planning subsequent surgical management. In the majority of patients a single primary fistula tract exists and the anatomy can be determined by examination under anaesthesia (EUA) adhering to the principles described by Goodsall. A thorough preoperative assessment with the patient awake is mandatory as sphincter length and integrity may be difficult to evaluate during anaesthesia. Asking the patient to voluntarily contract the external anal sphincter will demonstrate the levator plate and the anorectal junction. The lower border of the internal anal sphincter and intersphincteric groove can also be palpated and an estimation of internal and external anal sphincter length obtained. The external anal sphincter is deficient in the anterior upper third of the anal canal and may lead to a significantly shorter functional sphincter than would be expected by palpation of purely the posterior sphincter. The location of the external and internal opening or openings should be determined, and the primary tract can usually be palpated as a fibrous cord in the perianal area. Induration may be found in the anal canal at the site of the internal opening and on palpation of the tract pus may be expressed. Induration in the pararectal space is suggestive of supralevator extension of a primary or secondary tract. In some instances the use of high-resolution anorectal manometry can be useful in assessing preoperative sphincter function and length. This may aid decision making about whether fistulotomy may be safely performed.

Key Points

- A thorough clinical examination of the patient whilst awake and under general anaesthesia is essential in the assessment of fistula-in-ano.
- Determination of sphincter length, integrity and function is mandatory prior to consideration of fistulotomy.

IMAGING

The role of imaging is to assist with the identification of complex fistulous tracts and attempt to accurately define the anatomical relationship of the tracts to the anal sphincter muscles. This is thought to allow greater accuracy in surgical drainage and enables the surgeon to assess the potential risk of sphincter injury. Magnetic resonance imaging (MRI) and endo-anal ultrasonography are the most commonly used modalities. Recent meta-analysis however concluded that whilst imaging demonstrates adequate sensitivity in the detection of fistula, the specificity is diagnostically poor and gains little information over that observed during EUA.[3] Further studies are required to clarify the utility of these radiological tools.

Serial MRI may play a more important role in assessing outcomes of medical therapy in the treatment of Crohn's fistulae with anti-TNF agents. The EUA allows the use of fistula probes or hydrogen peroxide infiltrated into the tract to aid identification of the internal opening. The presence of secondary tracts is more difficult to evaluate and in some cases, if the anatomy is unclear, radiological assessment may be required to aid diagnosis. In the majority of simple fistulae however, radiological evaluation is not required.

> **Key Point**
>
> - Magnetic resonance imaging has poor specificity in defining the relationship of anal fistula tracts and should only be used in patients with complex fistulae in whom the anatomy is unclear during EUA.

CLASSIFICATION

Once the relationship of the fistula tract to the internal and external sphincters is established, the type of fistula can be documented using Parks' classification. Fistulae may be classified as high or low based on the amount of sphincter that lies below the tract. Traditionally, based on anatomical texts the dentate (pectinate) line lies at the junction between the lower one third and upper two-thirds of the anal canal and thus a fistula originating at or below this line is termed a low anal fistula (<30% sphincter involvement).

INITIAL TREATMENT

The goal of all fistula management is to control the sepsis and if possible, eradicate the tract whilst minimising the risk of faecal incontinence and recurrence. Fistulae may cause minimal symptoms or incapacitating pain and discharge and management has to be tailored to the patient taking into account the severity of their symptoms and their willingness to tolerate their symptoms or risk incontinence.

After defining the anatomy of the fistula tract or tracts, traditionally the initial goal of management has been to drain any sepsis and when possible eradicate the tract via fistulotomy, fistulectomy or a combination of both. Whilst many authors deem the laying open of low anal fistulae to be "safe", anatomical variation between patients needs to be considered. In some patients the sphincter is very short (<1 cm) and caution should be adopted, especially in female patients with anterior fistula tracts.

The risk of faecal incontinence increases with the complexity of the fistula. The more sphincter muscle included in the fistulotomy the higher the risk of incontinence.[4] In one large retrospective study, the risk of incontinence after fistulotomy for intersphincteric and trans-sphincteric fistulae was 37% and 54%, respectively, with higher rates seen with suprasphincteric and extrasphincteric fistulae.[5] Females are more likely to develop impaired continence following surgery when compared to males because of the shorter sphincter complex.[5] The risk of incontinence may be lower in those for whom the EAS is not divided.[6]

Whilst fistulotomy is the most effective cure for fistula-in-ano, if it cannot be safely performed then a loose seton is often placed. In the case of a transsphincteric fistula the external component of the tract can be laid open or excised to the external anal sphincter in an attempt to reduce pain and aid drainage. The implication and risks of more advanced surgical procedures can then be discussed with the patient before proceeding with any further intervention. Some patients will be content with a loose seton as acceptable definitive long-term management. In others, especially those with Crohns, this may be the preferred clinical option if the risk of incontinence or recurrence is high.

Cutting setons cause patient discomfort and appear not to eliminate the risk of incontinence and therefore are now seldom used. As many as two thirds of patients develop incontinence to flatus or liquid stool and one third to solid stool after use of a cutting seton, although this may reflect the complexity of the fistula for which the seton is used to treat.[7,8]

Key Point

- A loose seton can be an acceptable long-term treatment for patients who do not wish to risk incontinence resulting from surgical intervention to the anal sphincters.

ADVANCED TREATMENTS

Simple fistulae are effectively treated by fistulotomy. Advanced treatments are developed to deal with complex tracts (Flowchart 9.1). Complex fistula surgery often involves staged procedures if more than one third of the sphincter muscle is involved or there are multiple external orifices. The initial operation is often insertion of a loose seton to allow drainage and control infection.

The emphasis of recent advances in surgical technique has been to primarily eradicate the source of ongoing infection by isolation of the tract from the anal canal and removal of granulation tissue from the chronic epithelialised lining of the tract whilst minimising trauma to the sphincter muscles (sphincter-sparing measures). Treatments can be classified into those that aim to fill the fistula tract, those that aim to ligate the tract and those that aim to eradicate the tract via an endoluminal approach. Reported

Flowchart 9.1: Flowchart to show the current treatment options used for complex fistula-in-ano where a long-term seton or fistulotomy is deemed to be an unacceptable solution.

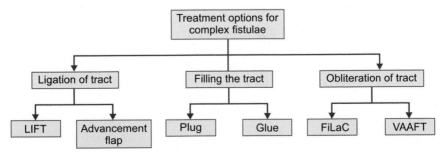

benefits of most treatments are derived from uncontrolled case studies that report retrospectively on only short-term outcomes. In many cases, heterogenicity of fistula type and aetiology makes comparison of different treatment modalities difficult. Smoking, diabetes and obesity appear to adversely affect the outcome of complex fistula surgery.

FILLING THE TRACT

Two treatments, glues and plugs, are simple to use, relatively inexpensive, and can be repeated, which may improve success rate (Table. 9.1).

Many clinicians advocate their use before other more invasive surgeries as they avoid the risk of incontinence, and create minimal stress for the patient.

Glues

Fibrin glue is the most popular compound used. This biological glue, made of fibrinogen, thrombin and other clotting factors, is injected into a prepared anal fistula tract in an attempt to seal it. Although numerous small, uncontrolled studies appear encouraging, meta-analysis has confirmed that healing only occurs in 50–60% of patients.[9,10] Results appear to be better when the glue is used in patients with simple fistulae.[10] A study performed by Singer, which considered antibiotics mixed in with fibrin glue, demonstrated no difference in healing rate.[11] Although healing at the external opening often is witnessed, only a small proportion of patients achieve clinical or radiological healing.[12] Future advances may relate to adding stem cells to the glue to help accelerate healing. In a randomized controlled trial comparing glue versus glue and stem cells in patients with cryptoglandular and Crohns fistulae, the use of stem cells appeared to significantly increase the rate and success of healing. Recurrence however still occurred in some patients in the medium term.[13] Further data are required to support the use of this expensive treatment prior to utilisation in routine practice.

Anal Fistula Plug

The anal fistula plug is made up of synthetic polymers that provide a scaffold to promote tract healing using a sphincter-preserving approach. It is positioned from inside the anus with sutures and conforms to the tract. A mucosal flap can be raised and used to cover the internal opening. There is wide variation in the reported effectiveness of fistula plugs although systematic review suggests that the proportion of patients achieving closure is likely to be in the region of 55% in both cryptoglandular and Crohn's fistulae.[14] Although a loose seton is often placed prior to a staged plug insertion, Chan et al. found that a successful outcome was more likely achieved in patient in whom no previous intervention had been performed.[15]

Table 9.1: Summary of clinical studies assessing the outcome of anal fistula plugs and glue in the treatment of fistula-in-ano.

Author	Year	Study Design	Method	Number of patients	Aetiology	Follow up (months)	Success rate (%)
Blom et al.	2014	PS	Biodesign plug	126	Complex cryptoglandular/crohn's	Median 13	24
Adamina et al.	2014	PS	Surgisis pulg	46	Complex cryptoglandular	Median 68	48
Tan et al.	2013	PS	Surgisis pulg	30	Cryptoglandular	Median 14	18%
Ommer et al.	2012	PS	Gore BioA Fistula plug	40	Complex cryptoglandular/crohn's	12	57.5
Swander et al.	2009	PS	Surgisis plug	60	Complex cryptoglandular	12	62
Thekkinkattil et al.	2009	PS	Surgisis plug	43	Complex cryptoglandular	Median 11	44
Safar et al.	2009	PS	Surgisis plug	35	Cryptoglandular/crohn's	Mean 4.2	13.9
Ky et al.	2008	PS	Surgisis plug	45	Cryptoglandular/ crohn's; simple & complex	Median 6.5	54.6
Champagne et al.	2006	PS	Surgisis plug	46	Complex cryptoglandular	Median 12	83
Christoforidis et al.	2009	Retrospective	Surgisis vs ERAF	43	Cryptoglandular	Mean 14 for plug	63 ERAF; 32 plug

Contd...

Contd...

Author	Year	Study Design	Method	Number of patients	Aetiology	Follow up (months)	Success rate (%)
De Parades	2012	PS	Fibrin glue	30	Complex cryptoglandular	1	50
Queralto et al.	2010	PS	Cyanoacrylate glue	34	Complex cryptoglandular	Median 34	67
Guadalajara et al.	2012	Retrospective	Fibrin glue +/- ASC's	34	Complex cryptoglandular/crohn's	Mean 43	33 ASC & glue; 15 glue
Han et al.	2011	Retrospective	Human acellular	114	Complex cryptoglandular	Median 19.5	54
Haim et al.	2011	PS	Fibrin glue	60	Complex cryptoglandular	Median 78	74
Van Koperan et al.	2011	RCT	Plug: ERAF	31:29	Complex cryptoglandular	11	29:48
Ortiz et al.	2009	RCT	Plug: ERAF	21:22	Complex cryptoglandular	12	
Ellix et al.	2006	RCT	ERAF: Fibrin glue	36:22	Complex cryptoglandular	Median	80 ERAF; 54

Table: Evidence summary of trials involving fistula plugs and glue; ASC's adipose derived stem cells; ERAF endorectal advancement flap; RCT randomized controlled trial; PS prospective case series;

Complications can include plug dislodgement, infection requiring drainage and/or seton placement, or failure with formation of a persistent tract. However, in those in whom the plug fails to close the tract, quality of life may still improve[16] and patients may have less persistent pain.[17] Risk factors for plug failure include smoking, diabetes or previous fistula surgery.

Key Points

- Fistula plugs and glue have a high failure rate with fistula healing occurring in only around one-half of patients.
- However, as their use does not preclude other treatments and the risk of sphincter damage is low they remain an attractive first-line surgical treatment option for tracts not amenable to fistulotomy.

LIGATION OF THE TRACT

Anorectal Advancement Flap

For many years anorectal advancement flaps have been used for high or complex anal fistulae where fistulotomy would otherwise have led to incontinence. The technique of advancement flap involves debridement of the fistula tract, utilisation of a well-vascularized rectal mucosal or anodermal flap to cover the internal opening of the tract with or without closure of the tract. The success rate at one year appears to be in the region of 60%.[18,19] Recent pilot data suggest that a similar outcome can be achieved by simply placing a super-elastic nitinol clip to occlude the internal opening, although larger studies with longer follow-up are required to see if this is a viable treatment option.[20]

Ligation of Intersphincteric Fistula Tract

Disconnection of the fistula tract from the anal canal with eradication or the tract in the intersphincteric space was first described in 1993.[21] It was not until recently however that ligation of the intersphincteric fistula tract (LIFT) gained popularity due to its reported success rate and low risk of incontinence. It is based on the concept of secure closure of the internal opening and concomitant removal of the infected cryptoglandular tissue in the intersphincteric plane.

The procedure involves a radial incision at the intersphincteric groove, with dissection continued cranially in the interspincteric plane to isolate the fistula tract as it crosses from the internal to the external sphincter. The tract is ligated with absorbable suture at the lateral border of the internal anal sphincter and the external component is treated by curettage or fistulotomy. Despite being known as a sphincter-sparing technique, it can involve a large amount of tissue dissection and in patients in whom previous surgery has been performed fibrosis and scarring can make the tract difficult to define. The technique seems most suited for patients with simple high trans-sphincteric fistulae of cryptoglandular aetiology and the majority of publications reporting the outcomes of the technique reflect this.[22] The role of a placing a pre-LIFT seton to control sepsis prior to performing the LIFT procedure remains unclear with little evidence of any beneficial role.[23]

Systematic review of the literature reports marked variation in clinical healing rates (40–95% success), which may reflect variations in surgical technique used.[22,23] Virtually, all studies report only short-term outcomes and use external opening closure to define healing without imaging to look for deeper eradication of sepsis. Pooled results suggest that in the short-term the clinical success rate of LIFT is 71–76%.[22,23] Modifications of the LIFT technique may yield higher success rates. Placement of a biological graft to reinforce the ligation and closure of the fistula tract, "BioLIFT",[24] has a reported success of fistula healing in 92% of patients. This is further reinforced with a study that used an anal plug to close the external tract in addition to the LIFT procedure.[25] This reported a 95% success rate, and a complete healing time of four weeks, faster than reported in other studies. The addition of a partial fistulotomy may also be beneficial with reported healing rates of 85% and no episodes of incontinence.[26]

Lehmann and Graf looked specifically at outcomes of LIFT performed for recurrent fistulae. The complete healing rate was 47%, with a persistence or recurrence of the fistula in 40% of patients.[27] One explanation for the lower cure rate may be due to fibrosis and scarring from chronic inflammation and previous interventions, which may result in obliteration of the intersphincteric space, thus making the tract difficult to identify and the dissection challenging.

Key Points

- The LIFT appears to be an attractive treatment option in the treatment of cryptoglandular trans-sphincteric fistulae with around three quarters of patients having successful healing.
- The results may not be as favourable when the technique is used for complex or recurrent fistulae.

OBLITERATION OF THE TRACT

Whilst not currently used in routine clinical practice, pilot studies have suggested that intra-luminal obliteration of the internal epithelialised surface of the fistula tract using diathermy or laser may be successful with minimal risk of sphincter damage. These techniques are experimental and their use should be monitored within a trial setting.

Video-assisted anal fistula treatment (VAAFT) uses a small 5-mm fistulo-scope, irrigation and diathermy to destroy the tract wall under direct vision with closure of the internal opening by stapler, suture or advancement flap. The only large study of 98 patients with predominantly trans-sphincteric fistulae reported a primary healing rate of 74% at three months.[28]

Fistula Laser Closure (FiLaC) uses a radial emitting laser probe, drawn through a prepared tract, which destroys the epithelial lining with mini-mal thermal spread or extra-luminal tissue damage. The internal opening is closed by advancement flap. Pilot data suggest a 71% closure rate at median 20 months follow-up with no reported deterioration in continence.[29]

Key Points

- Endoluminal obliteration of the fistula tract using Laser (FiLaC) or dia-thermy (VAAFT) is a novel approach in the treatment of fistulae with encouraging results in pilot data.
- Further well-designed prospective studies are required before these interventions are adopted into routine clinical practice.

CONCLUSION

In the last five years, there have been several new techniques developed to expedite the healing rates of anal fistulae whilst trying to maintain conti-nence. The LIFT procedure appears to be promising with high healing rates, low recurrence rates and minimal incontinence issues. The new endolu-minal eradication therapies (VAAFT and FiLaC) show promise, although there is currently a lack of efficacy data to support their use. It remains to be seen whether further randomised comparative trials with larger numbers of patients and longer follow-up will reveal similar favourable results. There is a trend to combine operative techniques, and one could speculate that further refinement of techniques will result in higher healing rates. Indeed, combining multiple approaches, including the use of biological agents (anti-TNF) to treat a fistula tailored on aetiology, anatomy and complexity, may yield the best results in the future.

For the patient, fistula surgery will always involve weighing-up what is an acceptable balance between risk of recurrence and risk of incontinence. Despite all the recent advances in surgical treatment, with each approach having advantages and disadvantages, fistulotomy still remains the gold standard in terms of cure, whereas the simple loose seton still has an impor-tant role to play in the management of complex fistulae.

REFERENCES

1. van Onkelen RS, et al. Assessment of microbiota and peptidoglycan in perianal fistulas. Diagn Microbiol Infect Dis. 2013;75(1):50-4.

2. Vasilevsky CA, Gordon PH. The incidence of recurrent abscesses or fistula-in-ano following anorectal suppuration. Dis Colon Rectum. 1984;27(2):126-30.
3. Siddiqui MR, et al. A diagnostic accuracy meta-analysis of endoanal ultrasound and MRI for perianal fistula assessment. Dis Colon Rectum. 2012;55(5):576-85.
4. Bokhari S, Lindsey I. Incontinence following sphincter division for treatment of anal fistula. Colorectal Dis. 2010;12(7 Online):e135-9.
5. Garcia-Aguilar J, et al. Anal fistula surgery. Factors associated with recurrence and incontinence. Dis Colon Rectum. 1996;39(7):723-9.
6. Kennedy HL, Zegarra JP. Fistulotomy without external sphincter division for high anal fistulae. Br J Surg, 1990;77(8):898-901.
7. Hamalainen KP, Sainio AP. Cutting seton for anal fistulas: high risk of minor control defects. Dis Colon Rectum. 1997;40(12):1443-6; discussion 1447.
8. Garcia-Aguilar J, et al. Cutting seton versus two-stage seton fistulotomy in the surgical management of high anal fistula. Br J Surg. 1998;85(2):243-5.
9. Cirocchi R, et al. Fibrin glue in the treatment of anal fistula: a systematic review. Ann Surg Innov Res. 2009;3:12.
10. Jacob TJ, Perakath B, Keighley MR. Surgical intervention for anorectal fistula. Cochrane Database Syst Rev,2010(5):CD006319.
11. Singer M, et al. Treatment of fistulas-in-ano with fibrin sealant in combination with intra-adhesive antibiotics and/or surgical closure of the internal fistula opening. Dis Colon Rectum. 2005;48(4):799-808.
12. Buchanan GN, et al. Efficacy of fibrin sealant in the management of complex anal fistula: a prospective trial. Dis Colon Rectum. 2003;46(9):1167-74.
13. Garcia-Olmo D, et al. Expanded adipose-derived stem cells for the treatment of complex perianal fistula: a phase II clinical trial. Dis Colon Rectum. 2009; 52(1):79-86.
14. O'Riordan JM, et al. A systematic review of the anal fistula plug for patients with Crohn's and non-Crohn's related fistula-in-ano. Dis Colon Rectum. 2012; 55(3):351-8.
15. Chan S, et al. Initial experience of treating anal fistula with the Surgisi anal fistula plug. Tech Coloproctol. 2012;16(3):201-6.
16. Adamina M, et al. Anal fistula plug: a prospective evaluation of success, continence and quality of life in the treatment of complex fistulae. Colorectal Dis. 2014;16(7):547-54.
17. Leng Q, Jin HY. Anal fistula plug vs mucosa advancement flap in complex fistula-in-ano: a meta-analysis. World J Gastrointest Surg. 2012;4(11):256-61.
18. Mizrahi N, et al. Endorectal advancement flap: are there predictors of failure? Dis Colon Rectum. 2002;45(12):1616-21.
19. van Onkelen RS, et al. Predictors of outcome after transanal advancement flap repair for high transsphincteric fistulas. Dis Colon Rectum. 2014;57(8):1007-11.
20. Prosst RL, Joos AK, Ehni W, et al. Prospective pilot study of anorectal fistula closure with the OTSC Proctology [published online ahead of print Sep 1, 2014]. Colorectal Dis.
21. Matos D, Lunniss PJ, Phillips RK. Total sphincter conservation in high fistula in ano: results of a new approach. Br J Surg. 1993;80(6):802-4.
22. Yassin NA, et al. Ligation of the intersphincteric fistula tract in the management of anal fistula. A systematic review. Colorectal Dis. 2013;15(5):527-35.
23. Hong KD, et al. Ligation of intersphincteric fistula tract (LIFT) to treat anal fistula: systematic review and meta-analysis. Tech Coloproctol. 2014;18(8):685-91.

24. Ellis CN. Outcomes with the use of bioprosthetic grafts to reinforce the ligation of the intersphincteric fistula tract (BioLIFT procedure) for the management of complex anal fistulas. Dis Colon Rectum. 2010;53(10):1361-4.

25. Han JG, et al. Ligation of the intersphincteric fistula tract plus a bioprosthetic anal fistula plug (LIFT-Plug): a new technique for fistula-in-ano. Colorectal Dis. 2013;15(5):582-6.

26. Sirikurnpiboon S, Awapittaya B, Jivapaisarnpong P. Ligation of intersphincteric fistula tract and its modification: Results from treatment of complex fistula. World J Gastrointest Surg, 2013;5(4):123-8.

27. Lehmann JP, Graf W. Efficacy of LIFT for recurrent anal fistula. Colorectal Dis. 2013;15(5):592-5.

28. Meinero P, Mori L. Video-assisted anal fistula treatment (VAAFT): a novel sphincter-saving procedure for treating complex anal fistulas. Tech Coloproctol. 2011;15(4):417-22.

29. Giamundo P. et al. Closure of fistula-in-ano with laser--FiLaC: an effective novel sphincter-saving procedure for complex disease. Colorectal Dis. 2014;16(2): 110-5.

10
Chapter

The Use of Robotics in Colorectal Surgery

Arifa Siddika, Shahab Siddiqui

HISTORY OF ROBOTIC SURGERY

Heartthrob was the world's first surgical robot and performed the first ever robotic operation, an arthroscopy, in Vancouver in 1984. Further developments included the Unimation Puma 200 robot used to place a CT-guided needle for a brain biopsy in 1985,[1] PROBOT with the world first pure robotic operation on a prostate at Guy's and St Thomas' Hospital, London, in 1992, and also in that year ROBODOC, which milled out precise fittings in the femur for hip replacement.[2] SRI International developed robotic systems further with the help of grants from NASA.[3] The first robotic surgery using this system was performed in Ohio, USA, followed by a variety of procedures; fallopian tube reconnection in 1998, a beating heart coronary artery bypass graft in 1999[4] and a cholecystectomy performed remotely in 2001.

Intuitive Surgical bought the patents from SRI International and these allowed the da Vinci robots to sense the surgeon's hand movements and then translate them electronically into scaled-down micromovements to manipulate the robotic instruments. Other features detect and filter out physiological tremor in the surgeon's hand movements and the use of two cameras allow a true stereoscopic picture to be transmitted to the surgeon's console.[5] Milestones for the da Vinci system include a heart bypass in Germany in 1998 and the first all-robotic-assisted kidney transplant in 2009. The da Vinci Si was released in 2009 and had an option of dual surgeon consoles to facilitate training.[6] The patents bought from SRI International are due to expire in 2015 and 2016. Since then robotic surgery has evolved in most fields of surgery, but radical prostatectomy remains the most widely performed and accepted robotic operation.[7,8]

ROBOTIC SURGERY— ADVANTAGES AND DISADVANTAGES

Robotic surgery has many advantages of minimally invasive surgery. Instrument articulation beyond normal laparoscopic (or even human) manipulation and three-dimensional magnification results in improved ergonomics and precision. Additionally, the camera view does not deteriorate with assistant fatigue or inexperience. There are many reports that show robotic surgery to be comparable to laparoscopic and open surgery in terms of outcome.[9,10] Learning curves are said to be less than laparoscopic approaches and surgeons report less fatigue. However, only one operation has proved its effectiveness above its laparoscopic and open counterparts, namely robotic radical prostatectomy. The 3D view and instrument manipulation allow visualisation and protection of the pelvic nerves to an unmatched degree. Operations in fixed small spaces with the inherent poor access, such as oral and pelvic surgery, have benefited from the fixed robotic platform. The ergonomics and precision make intracorporeal suturing far easier than laparoscopic. New technologies also allow the assessment of bowel vascularity prior to anastomosis.[11] The progress is more evolution than revolution.

Robotic surgery has pitfalls, but this is expected for early generation technology. The slave robot unit arms needs to be connected (docked) with the trocars placed in the patient. In colorectal surgery, this entails an initial laparoscopy (the robot camera can be used to save costs, but is heavy) with placement of the appropriate ports. These ports are currently wider and more numerous than the corresponding ports needed for the equivalent laparoscopic operation and need to be placed carefully.

For all colorectal procedures a reverse Trendelenburg position is needed with appropriate patient protection. Once ports are placed and small bowel moved out of the operative field, the slave robot unit is moved by an assistant to the patient side. This is known as docking with the camera, target and slave unit that need to be in a straight line. End docking between the legs is easiest, with least robot arm clashing, but limits access to the perineum. Side docking is more flexible, but can lead to more clashing of the arms. Once docked further patient movement is not possible without de-docking the slave unit. This means that splenic flexure mobilisation is completed in this position rather than the usual head-up position used in laparoscopy. This restricted movement is more important if the patient becomes acutely unwell and the anaesthetist demands an immediate halt to the surgery and needs the patient be placed supine with the removal of all instruments. It is therefore essential that emergency de-docking be discussed at stage 2 of World Health Organisation check single time and practiced regularly. The lack of tactile (haptic) feedback can be overcome by developing and recognising surrogate markers of tension. Surgery for robotic surgeons is much more visual based.

Early in the learning curve, robot arm clashing can be frustrating and limiting. Once the system is understood, this becomes more limited and less of a problem especially when compared to a difficult low rectal cancer case performed laparoscopically where clashing does limit dissection.[12] Recent robot technology was designed for one-quadrant surgery, which is fine for certain surgical specialties, but not colorectal surgery. Surgeons were pragmatic and used hybrid techniques (laparoscopic abdominal and pelvic robotic surgery), dual robot docking and single robot docking techniques to overcome this limitation.[9] Newer technology will aid this also.

The robotic system is expensive to purchase and maintain. The da Vinci series costs a million pounds or more and its disposable supply cost is £1,000 per case.[10] The instruments are reusable, but restricted to 10 different cases. After an instrument has been utilised in 10 different patients, the robot will not accept its further use irrespective of the total time each instrument has been used. This leads to the situation where some instruments are used for more than 30 hours and others for 30 minutes after their use in 10 patients, but both cost £3,000. Interestingly, Intuitive Surgical allows the same instruments to be used up to 30 times in some countries. It is expected that the current UK limit will be raised as pressure from competitors mounts. There is a shelf life to each robotic system (five to seven years), but the trade-in values are high.

An additional tariff is chargeable with robotic procedures in the NHS. NHS England is reviewing the evidence for each different surgical procedure and if not supported may allow local Clinical Commissioning Groups to pay the lesser laparoscopic tariff. This may add to the many hospital trusts looking to end their robotic programs especially if they do not operate on prostate cancer, which already has the support of NICE. With the current tight fiscal demands on the NHS, NHS England has placed a moratorium on new robot system purchases. Although cost-effectiveness is difficult to calculate, it seems that 150–250 cases need to be done annually to make each robotic system cost-effective.[7] This may require changes in job plans and theatre utilisation. Additional cost pressures come from the fact that operative time for robotic operations is generally longer.[8]

The initial take-up of robotic surgery was reminiscent of the take-up of laparoscopic cholecystectomy. Individuals took on the challenge, some without the appropriate training leading to an excess of complications, off-camera injuries and deaths.[12] This has led to the statement made by the President of the American College of Obstetric and Gynecology earlier this year warning of the wide-scale adoption of robotic surgery, surgeons jumping on the robotic bandwagon and the lack of evidence.[13]

Multiple litigations claims are pending against Intuitive Surgical in the United States. Partly because of this, training for robotic surgery is becoming more formalised not only for the surgeon but also for the whole team.[11] This has come from the industry as well as the clinical governance structure in hospital trusts. The learning phase is intensive and it is recommended that surgeons must operate on 12–18 patients before they adapt to robotic operating. During the training phase, the procedures can take up to twice as long as traditional surgery, leading to reallocation of resources and prolonged anaesthesia for patients. Accreditation may additionally be needed in individual operations.

Key Points

- Robot-assisted surgery has overcome some of the limitations of minimal access surgery.
- Robotic systems provide unparalleled 3D views, precise dissection and a stable operating base.
- Robotic surgery has disadvantages such as greater cost, longer operative time, lack of haptic feedback and limited intra-quadrant manoeuvrability.
- Various bodies are now working on training and accreditation for robotic colorectal surgery.

COLORECTAL SURGERY

The colorectal world has been slow to take up robotic surgery. However, there are now several series published which include over a thousand patients, mostly from South Korea and the United States.[14] Results to date indicate that robotic-assisted colorectal procedures are safe and outcomes are comparable to laparoscopic or open surgery. In fact some studies indicate better outcome in terms of reduced pain, decreased length of hospital stay and quicker recovery.[15] Most of the studies have been for colon and rectal cancer, but a few include benign disease. The vast majority of the studies use the da Vinci robots.

Right Hemicolectomy

Various series were published for early results of right hemicolectomy confirming feasibility, safety and equivalent outcome.[15,16] Advantages of a robotic approach are the increased precision of dissection and option of an easier intracorporeal anastomosis. However, there are major disadvantages—e.g. prolonged duration of surgery, increased cost and the one-quadrant nature of the da Vinci—which actually may make the surgery more difficult.[16]

A standard laparoscopic right hemicolectomy is not a challenging procedure, with good results. It is of no surprise that there is decreasing interest in performing this procedure robotically, and most robotic colorectal surgeons prefer the laparoscopic approach to the robotic approach. This preference may change with improving technology.

Anterior Resection

A narrow pelvis can be a surgical challenge, but this is where robotic colorectal surgery has its greatest potential. Anterior resection is the commonest robotic colorectal operation performed.[16] It does not make a difficult pelvis easy, but can be a definite advantage. The 3D image and enhanced vision help identify the pelvic nerves accurately, and the articulated robotic instruments allow precise dissection.

Anterior resection is a three-quadrant operation and the original da Vinci robots were not designed for this without intraoperative re-docking. As such, there are many ways to perform an anterior resection. Hybrid techniques involve laparoscopic abdominal surgery and robotic pelvic surgery.[17] There are several ways to perform a completely robotic anterior resection. Duel docking techniques involve one docking for the splenic flexure and another for the remainder. Single docking anterior resection involves a solitary docking in the left iliac fossa, but still requires the robot arms to be shifted to different trocars when moving from the abdominal to the pelvic section of the procedure.[18] The surgical technique uses conventional laparoscopic medial to lateral mobilisation; however, the robotic ports' placement is completely differently compared to the laparoscopic technique (Figs. 10.1 to 10.3).

The major advantage of the robotic technique is the precision of dissection, which gives a better total mesorectal excision with reduced pelvic nerve damage. A systemic analysis suggested that oncological outcomes are comparable if not better with the use of a robot.[10] However, there are some well-recognised disadvantages such as increased operating time, longer learning curve, increased cost, lack of tactile feedback and lack of overall view.

European accreditation for low anterior section has been launched in October 2014 led by the Portsmouth group. It involves a standardised single docking methodology. Only two to three groups in the UK perform single docking anterior resections at present so it remains to be seen if other units will adopt this as well.

ROLARR and SOLARR are international randomised trials comparing laparoscopic and robotic rectal cancer surgery. The results are eagerly

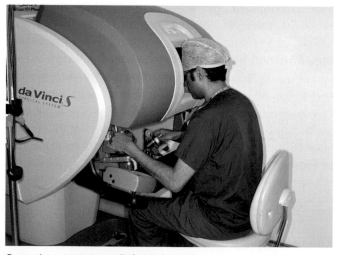

Fig. 10.1: Operating surgeon at Robotic console.

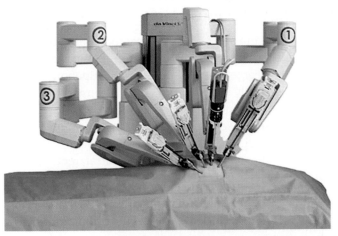

Fig. 10.2: Schematic view of robot slave unit with docked arms without sterile drapes.

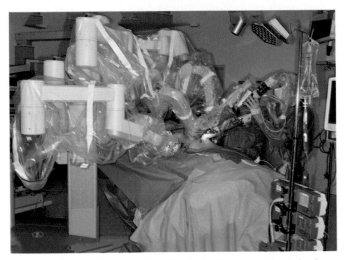

Fig. 10.3: Patient side robot slave unit with docked arms and sterile drapes.

awaited, but doubts remain about the lack of standardised robotic operative methodology. As long as the pelvic surgery was done robotically it was accepted into the trials.[19,20]

Key Points

- Various bodies are now working on training and accreditation for robotic colorectal surgery.
- Low anterior resection and ventral mesh rectopexy are the commonest colorectal operations performed.

SURGERY FOR INTERNAL AND EXTERNAL RECTAL PROLAPSE

Laparoscopic ventral mesh rectopexy and sacrocolporectopexy have become the gold standard for both internal and external rectal prolapse since they result in the least degree of postoperative constipation and recurrence.[21] Robotic surgery is ideally suited for this type of surgery. The 3D views, precision of dissection and incorporeal suturing allow surgery not achievable laparoscopically. Various series have shown results similar to that found in larger laparoscopic series.

Most laparoscopic techniques involve ventral rectal dissection only. Robotic surgery allows this as well. However, as one can dissect extensively down the narrow anterior dissection tube, this allows the pelvic floor to be exposed widely once beyond the important pelvic nerves. This enables the ventral mesh to be sutured to the pelvic floor as well as to the rectum.

Ventral mesh rectopexy for internal rectal prolapse has a recurrence rate, half of which comes from a large posterior internal prolapse that has not been dealt with sufficiently. The Oxford Pelvic Floor Group suggested a limited posterior dissection and mesh for certain patients at higher risk of failure in addition to the ventral mesh. Posterior dissection risks postoperative constipation especially if dissection is too lateral. Limited posterior dissection still requires mesh to be sutured to mesorectal fat that is not ideal for fixation. Robotic modified Orr-Loygue involves a standard ventral mesh plus a narrow mesh posteriorly. Robotic dissection allows a long narrow tube to be dissected posterior to the rectum, in between the hypogastric nerves down to the rectal tube and Waldeyer's fascia allowing mesh to be sutured to the rectal muscle.[22-26] It is not yet known whether this improves outcome.

The disadvantages of this technique are as with any robotic surgical technique, increased cost, prolonged surgery and off sight injury.

Transanal Surgery

One can perform single access surgery with certain types of da Vinci robot. This would mean TEMS/TAMIS/TASER-type procedures could be performed with all the visual and suturing advantages of the robotic platform.[6]

Total Colectomy

At present the transverse colon remains too flexible an organ to deal with robotically.

FUTURE DEVELOPMENTS

Intuitive Surgical's share price is at an all-time high, but profits are low especially when compared to the turnover. This has analysts worried for several reasons. The patents for many of the da Vinci robots run out 2015/6 with competitors now appearing on the market. The new da Vinci robot Xi is a spectacular machine, but despite it costing the same as the current da Vinci robot, technology experts are disappointed with it. The Xi has been designed for multi-quadrant work, with arms that automatically deploy in positions to avoid clashing. The robot also swings round to make a total colectomy possible. The problem with the Xi is that its competitors are based on a single incision/access system and cost less than half the price. Another dark cloud on the horizon for Intuitive Surgical is the pending litigations that have the potential to derail the company.

Single access,[27] multi-quadrant robotic surgery, with costs far closer to laparoscopic counterparts, is a mouth-watering prospect and does not seem that far off. Current da Vinci robots are early generation machines. If surgical robotic technology goes the way of other technology such as smart phones, then nearly every abdominal operation will be possible using a robot. However, if there is a mushrooming of different robots and technologies, then training will become a major problem with its subsequent effect on patient safety.

Key Points

- Robotic surgery has already surpassed what is achievable laparoscopically.
- Even the limited number of procedures performed, studies have already shown robotic surgery to be at least the equivalent of laparoscopic and open surgery.
- Newer generation robots promise greatly improved functionality, single incision multi-quadrant access with markedly reduced cost may make robotic surgery widely acceptable.

REFERENCES

1. Meadows M. Computer-assisted surgery: an update. FDA Consumer Magazine. Food and Drug Administration. Available from http://www.fda.gov/fdac/features (accessed 25 September 14).
2. McConnell PI, Schneeberger EW, Michler RE. History and development of robotic cardiac surgery. Prob Gen Surg. 2003;20(2):20-30.
3. Robotics: the Future of Minimally Invasive Heart Surgery. Available from http://Biomed.brown.edu/courses/bi108 (accessed 27 September 14).
4. Gerhardus D. Robot-assisted surgery: the future is here. J Healthc Manag. 2003;48(4):242-51.
5. da Vinci Si Surgical System. Intuitive Surgical. Available from http://intutivesurgical.com/products (accessed 22 September 14).
6. Ramsay C, Pickard R, Robertson C, et al. Systematic review and economic modelling of the relative clinical benefit and cost-effectiveness of laparoscopic surgery and robotic surgery for removal of the prostate in men with localised prostate cancer. Health Technol Assess. 2012;16(41):1-313.
7. Sandoval Salinas C, Gonzalez Rangel AL, Catano Catano JG, et al. Efficacy of robotic-assisted prostatectomy in localized prostate cancer: a systematic review of clinical trials. Adv Urol. 2013;2013:105651.

8. Liao G, Zhao Z, Lin S, et al. Robotic-assisted versus laparoscopic colorectal surgery: a meta-analysis of four randomized controlled trials. World J Surg Oncol. 2014;12:122.

9. Kim CW, Kim CH, Baik SH. Outcomes of robotic-assisted colorectal surgery compared with laparoscopic and open surgery: a systematic review. J Gastrointest Surg. 2014;18(4):816-30.

10. Hellan M, Spinoglio G, Pigazzi A, et al. The influence of fluorescence imaging on the location of bowel transection during robotic left-sided colorectal surgery. Surg Endosc. 2014;28(5):1695-702.

11. Wormer BA, Dacey KT, Williams KB, et al. The first nationwide evaluation of robotic general surgery: a regionalized, small but safe start. Surg Endosc. 2014;28(3): 767-76.

12. http://www.acog.org/About-ACOG/News-Room/News-Releases/2013/Statement-on-Robotic-Surgery (accessed on 28 September 2014).

13. Aly EH. Robotic colorectal surgery: summary of the current evidence. Int J Colorectal Dis. 2014;29(1):1-8.

14. deSouza AL, Prasad LM, Park JJ, et al. Robotic assistance in right hemicolectomy: is there a role? Dis Colon Rectum. 2010;53(7):1000-6.

15. Mak TW, Lee JF, Futaba K, et al. Robotic surgery for rectal cancer: a systematic review of current practice. World J Gastrointest Oncol. 2014;6(6):184-93.

16. Morpurgo E, Contardo T, Molaro R, et al. Robotic-assisted intracorporeal anastomosis versus extracorporeal anastomosis in laparoscopic right hemicolectomy for cancer: a case control study. J Laparoendosc Adv Surg Tech A. 2013;23(5): 414-7.

17. Zawadzki M, Velchuru VR, Albalawi SA, et al. Is hybrid robotic laparoscopic assistance the ideal approach for restorative rectal cancer dissection? Colorectal Dis. 2013;15(8):1026-32.

18. Kim SH, Kwak JM. Robotic total mesorectal excision: operative technique and review of the literature. Tech Coloproctol. 2013;17(1):S47-53.

19. http://ctru.leeds.ac.uk/rolarr.

20. http://clinicaltrials.gov/ct2/show/NCT01736072.

21. Germain A, Perrenot C, Scherrer ML, et al. Long-term outcome of robotic-assisted laparoscopic rectopexy for full-thickness rectal prolapse in elderly patients. Colorectal Dis. 2014;16(3):198-202.

22. Mantoo S, Podevin J, Regenet N, et al. Is robotic-assisted ventral mesh rectopexy superior to laparoscopic ventral mesh rectopexy in the management of obstructed defaecation? Colorectal Dis. 2013;15(8):469-75.

23. Kanji A, Gill RS, Shi X, et al. Robotic-assisted colon and rectal surgery: a systematic review. Int J Med Robot. 2011;7(4):401-7.

24. Patel CB, Ramos-Valadez DI, Haas EM. Robotic-assisted laparoscopic abdominoperineal resection for anal cancer: feasibility and technical considerations. Int J Med Robot. 2010;6(4):399-404.

25. Baek JH, McKenzie S, Garcia-Anguilar J, et al. Oncologic outcomes of robotic-assisted total mesorectal excision for the treatment of rectal cancer. Ann Surg. 2010;251(5):882-6.

26. Luca F, Cenciarelli S, Valvo M, et al. Full robotic left colon and rectal cancer resection: technique and early outcome. Ann Surg Oncol. 2009;16(5):1274-8.

27. Autorino R, Kaouk JH, Stolzenburg JU, et al. Current status and future directions of robotic single-site surgery: a systematic review. Eur Urol. 2013;63(2):266-80.

Section
4

Surgical
Oncology

11

Chapter

Modern Prostate Cancer Management

Taimur Shah, Manit Arya, John D Kelly

INTRODUCTION

In the United Kingdom over 40,000 new cases and over 10,000 deaths occur each year as a result of prostate cancer, making it the commonest cancer and second leading cause of cancer-related death in men. Fortunately, 80% of men will survive for at least five years after the initial diagnosis.

The incidence of prostate cancer increases with age and postmortem data demonstrates histological prostate cancer in approximately 30% of all men in their 40s and in up to 90% of men in their 80s–90s. However, the actual clinical incidence peaks at age 65–79 but then drops thereafter, which may be due to a lower rate of prostate-specific antigen (PSA) testing in this older population. The lifetime risk of developing prostate cancer in the United Kingdom is 1 in 8.

SCREENING

The multi-centre European Randomized Study of Screening for Prostate Cancer (ERSPC) was established in 1994 in which 162,388 men aged 55–69 were randomised to either receive PSA-based screening or not, with an 11-year follow-up.[1]

It is the only study to show a significant benefit from screening with 0.4% of the patients assigned to PSA screening dying from prostate cancer, compared to 0.5% in the control group. No difference was seen in all-cause mortality.

To prevent one prostate cancer death the number needed to screen was 781 or one per 27 men diagnosed. Although this study showed a benefit for screening this needs to be balanced against overdiagnosis and subsequent overtreatment.

Not all agree with these findings and the results of 80,379 patients from the Finland section showed a non-significant decrease in mortality.[2] Attention has also focused on the Swedish section, which had a four times greater absolute survival benefit compared to the overall ERSPC results. In addition the Swedish section had a longer overall follow-up, included younger men (aged 50–54 years) and had an inappropriately high rate of primary androgen deprivation therapy (ADT) in the control arm.[3]

Another important study was the United States multi-centre Prostate, Lung, Colorectal and Ovarian cancer screening trial (PLCO).[4] A total of 76,693 men were randomised to either screening (PSA and DRE) or to standard care. Their updated data from 2012 showed that after 15 years of follow-up no significant difference in prostate cancer-specific mortality was seen between the two groups. These results were in stark contrast to the results from the ERSPC study. However, 44% of patients had undergone PSA testing prior to randomisation thus potentially eliminating aggressive disease and subsequently 52% of patients in the control arm had opportunistic screening, which may have led to significant contamination of the results.

A subsequent Cochrane review of five prostate cancer screening randomised control trials (RCTs) found no benefit to screening after a pooled meta-analysis.[5] They did comment that 3 out of the 5 studies had potential for a high level of bias whilst the ERSPC and PLCO studies had a low level of bias but had opposing results.

The United States preventative services task force (USPSTF) reviewed existing literature and updated their 2008 recommendations. In 2008, the USPSTF recommended against PSA testing in men aged ≥ 75 years and that there was inconclusive evidence for use in men aged 50–74 years. In 2011, the task force commented that the implications for healthcare have not yet been fully realized and they recommended that no healthy man should undergo PSA screening unless he has symptoms of prostate cancer.

The British Association of Urological Surgeons also does not currently recommend screening and the American Urological Association recommends screening in the 55–69 age groups only after an informed shared decision discussing potential benefits and risks has taken place.

Key Point

- The incidence of prostate cancer increases with age and post-mortem data demonstrates histological prostate cancer in approximately 30% of all men in their 40s and in up to 90% of men in their 80s–90s.

DIAGNOSIS

Transrectal Ultrasound-Guided Biopsies

Transrectal ultrasound-guided (TRUS) biopsy has been the staple prostate cancer diagnostic procedure for over two decades. A 7.5-MHz multiplanar probe is used to visualise the prostate and most commonly 10–12 cores are taken using a periprostatic block. This can be easily performed in an office or day case setting.

There have however been many criticisms of this technique. Analysis of radical prostatectomy specimens have found that 20–25% of patients may harbour anterior tumours, which can be missed by the transrectal approach.[6,7] In addition, over 30% of patients will be found to have a tumour after rebiopsy with a negative initial biopsy and persistent concern for prostate cancer. Another concern with TRUS biopsies has been an associated sepsis rate of up to 6% due to passage of the needle through rectal flora. Different antibiotic regimes have been implemented dependent on local antibiotic sensitivities.

Multiple methods have been described to improve the diagnostic yield of the prostate biopsy, which include transrectal saturation, transperineal (TP) saturation and most recently multi-parametric magnetic resonance imaging (mpMRI)-guided biopsies. A systematic review by Nelson et al. found no significant difference in yield between any of the three options with all finding cancer in approximately 30–40% of cases.[8] However, mpMRI-guided biopsies produced these results with significantly fewer cores taken per patient.

Transperineal Biopsies

Transperineal biopsies have been gaining popularity not only with a view to improve accuracy but also to reduce the risk of sepsis. The sepsis rate is <1%; however, acute urinary retention appears to be more common with TP biopsies and ranges from 2% to 9%.[9]

Barzell and Melamed have described a mapping TP technique by using a brachytherapy grid and sampling every 5 mm.[10] Onik et al. used this technique to assess patients for focal cryotherapy of the prostate and found that after taking a mean of 50 cores, 23% of cancers were upgraded whilst 60% of patients had bilateral disease.[11] Due to the sampling frame it is possible to miss tumours <5 mm and thus the diagnostic accuracy for clinically significant cancer is between 90% and 95% when compared to a radical prostatectomy specimens.

Multiparametric MRI

As mentioned mpMRI is a newly evolving technique. Initially, prebiopsy T2-weighted MRI was used to avoid post-biopsy haemorrhage artefacts within the prostate. This artefact may lead to difficulty in local diagnosis and staging and can take weeks to months to resolve.

Additional diffusion weighted and gadolinium dynamic contrast enhanced sequences (Fig. 11.1) were added to the standard T2-weighted sequences to develop mpMRI as a primary diagnostic tool, with biopsies only being taken if the mpMRI demonstrates a lesion. A 1.5 or 3 Tesla scanner is used along with either a pelvic-phased array or endorectal coil to improve on the signal-noise ratio and to improve spatial resolution. Diffusion weighting assesses the restriction in free movement of water

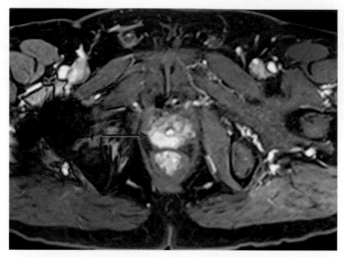

Fig. 11.1: Dynamic contrast-enhanced multiparametric magnetic resonance imaging prostate. Contrast-enhanced sequence demonstrating right peripheral zone tumour.

within cancerous tissue due to its cellular architecture, whereas contrast sequences assess the early perfusion of cancerous tissue due to angiogenesis.

A Likert scale is normally used from 1 to 5, which correlates well with the odds of detecting cancer.[12] Puech et al. compared mpMRI to radical retropubic prostatectomy (RRP) specimens and found that it had a diagnostic accuracy of 75%, largely due to a specificity of 95%.[13] Haffner et al. assessed whether only targeting MRI positive lesions was possible and found that targeted cores had an equal ability to pick up significant cancer when compared to standard 12 core TRUS biopsies, but with a mean of only 3.8 cores taken per patient.[14]

Ultrasound fusion techniques have also been developed to allow more accurate targeting of lesions. Siddiqui et al. performed a TRUS biopsy and MRI/ultrasound fusion targeted biopsy in 582 patients. The addition of a targeted biopsy led to an upgrading of tumour in 32% of patients. Fusion targeted biopsy detected 67% more Gleason >4+3 disease compared to TRUS and missed 36% of Gleason <3+4 thus potentially reducing the risk of over diagnosis.[15]

Overall, mpMRI appears to be here to stay but its exact role is yet to be established. Many studies have quoted a negative predictive value of between 80–90% for significant cancer, and this appears to give it an advantage in selecting patients for subsequent biopsy but currently data is only available from high volume centres and doubts exist on reproducibly in local hospitals.[12,16-18] Similarly, performing purely targeted biopsies raises concerns of missing significant disease and in the authors' opinion both standard and targeted biopsies will need to be performed to give the highest diagnostic yield and accuracy. Work is also underway in using mpMRI as a method for selection and follow-up of patients on active surveillance (AS) protocols.

Natural History of Prostate Cancer

Albertson followed up 767 patients for a median of 24 years who had a diagnosis of nonmetastatic prostate cancer made after either transurethral resection of prostate (TURP) (71%) or biopsy (26%) and were unable to have radical treatments. He found that untreated Gleason 6 disease had a cancer specific mortality (CSM) of 27%, whereas this was between 40% and 90% for Gleason >7 disease.[19] Data from the Scandinavian prostate cancer group-4 (SPCG-4) trial also showed that with watchful waiting (WW) 72% of patients with mainly clinically detected prostate cancer were alive after 23-year follow up.[20] From the hormone therapy arm of the SPCG-7 study where the majority of patients had T3 disease, the cancer-specific survival (CSS) was 76.1% at 10 years.[21]

Although on radical prostatectomy specimens prostate cancer is commonly multi-focal, some of these results may be explained by the fact that small volume tumours may be clinically insignificant. Similarly, re-review of Eggener et al's data on 9,554 patients showed a 0% mortality at 15 years in those with true Gleason 6 disease.[22] Ross et al. also showed that no lymph node metastases occurred in 14,000 radical prostatectomy and lymph node specimens of patients with Gleason 6 disease.[23]

Further work has shown that progression and metastases may be linked to an index lesion. Small volume Gleason 6 disease may not meet the criteria to be classified as a cancer whilst mice models have shown that only specific tumour lines are responsible for metastases. Human autopsy studies have also confirmed this mono-clonal origin for lethal disease.[24-26]

Thus, it is clear that not all prostate cancer is created equal and this needs to incorporated into discussions with patients regarding their management.

Key Points

- With WW 72% of patients with mainly clinically detected prostate cancer are alive after 23 years follow-up.
- From the hormone therapy arm of the SPCG-7 study where the majority of patients had T3 disease, the CSS was 76.1% at 10 years.

TREATMENT

The exact management strategy depends not only on the stage and grade of the disease but also on the patient's age, comorbidities and ultimately their preference. The most common options are AS, radical treatments such as RRP, external beam radiotherapy (EBRT), brachytherapy or focal treatments such as cryotherapy or high-intensity focused ultrasound (HIFU).

Active Surveillance

Active surveillance protocols were implemented in an attempt to defer radical treatment for patients and thus avoid their potential significant side effects. Different criteria exist for defining low-risk disease, which may be suitable for an initial surveillance strategy. The updated Epstien criteria from 2004 define low-risk disease as clinical stage < T1, no pattern 4, PSA density $\leq$ 0.15, $\leq$2 positive cores and <50% single core involvement.[27] Many series use this as their selection criteria for AS whilst others use the D'Amico low risk category and occasionally Gleason 3+4 disease is also included, such as in the Royal Marsden criteria.[28]

The longest running series is by Klotz with a median of 6.8 years of follow-up.[29] This series includes 450 patients of which 30% would be classified as moderate risk disease (Gleason 3+4 and PSA <15). The 10-year actuarial CSS was 97.2% with only five deaths noted. Overall, 30% of patients eventually ended up having radical treatment, most commonly due to reclassification of disease after biopsy for a PSA doubling time (PSADT) < 3 years. Similar results with an almost 100% CSS have been seen by others and the largest series of 988 patients of low-risk prostate cancer is taken from the ERSPC screening trial where estimated 10-year CSS is 100%.[30]

Most AS protocols also include a repeat biopsy and as we have already mentioned this can re-classify disease in approximately 30% of patients thus making them unsuitable for surveillance. The timing of this biopsy is variable but most commonly is performed at one year. Biopsies for progression are normally performed when PSADT < 3 years or if there is change in clinical stage.

The subsequent outcomes of patients undergoing radical treatment after a period of AS appear not to be compromised. Eighty-six per cent of the patients in Klotz's series remain untreated or without failure of secondary treatment.[29]

Radical Prostatectomy

Prior to wide spread PSA testing the SPGC-4 RCT compared WW with radical prostatectomy. A total of 695 men met the inclusion criteria of age < 75 years, clinical T1 or T2 disease, a life expectancy > 10 years, a PSA of < 50 and a negative bone scan. They were randomly assigned to have either an RRP or WW. Patients were reviewed six monthly for two years and then annually. Those on WW were allowed palliative or symptomatic treatment such as ADT or TURP.

The results have been updated and published on four occasions with 23 years of follow-up (median 13.4 years). The original results in 2005 paper showed an increased CSS of 5.8% in favour of RRP compared to WW (8.6% vs 14.4%). The overall mortality in those undergoing prostatectomy was 23.9% compared to 30.5% in those selected for WW, 83 versus 106 men respectively. This difference continued to increase over time and the 2014 data quotes a number needed to treat to prevent one death as 8. Those aged < 65 years had the greatest benefit with the number needed to treat being 4. In addition, RRP also conveys a reduction in metastases if performed in older men.[20,31-33]

In the PSA era a US study called the "Prostate Cancer Intervention Versus Observation Trial" has also attempted to determine whether there was any benefit to radical surgery in patients with prostate cancer. They randomised 731 men to compare radical prostatectomy against observation in localised prostate cancer. Fifty perent of men had T1c and after a median follow-up of 10 years no significant difference in either all cause or CSM was seen. However, subgroup analysis showed that in patients with a PSA > 10 ng/mL, radical prostatectomy was associated with a 7.2% reduction in CSM. They also showed trending data for a benefit in those with intermediate and high-risk disease.[34]

The opposing results in these two studies may be explained by the fact that they recruited patients at different stages of their disease. PSA screening has led to a stage migration with patients being detected with T1c, clinically impalpable disease compared with those who present with symptoms. Thus offering prostatectomy to low-risk patients may not have any benefit. However patients at higher risk such as those with a PSA >10 ng/mL and/or clinically palpable disease may have benefit from radical prostatectomy. Furthermore, retrospective and cohort reviews have shown that RRP carries better outcomes in high risk and locally advanced disease than other treatment options such as radiotherapy or hormone deprivation.

Comparing the surgical methods for robotic, laparoscopic or open radical prostatectomy, a significant difference in oncological outcomes has not been shown. Two series of over 1000 patients having RRPs have shown a 96% biochemical disease-free survival (bDFS) at one year, 90% at three years and 87% at five years.[35,36] Unsurprisingly, in patients with high-risk disease the outcomes are worse with a one year bDFS of 71% at dropping to 59% at three years.[37] Apart from a benefit to the surgeon robotic and laparoscopic procedures have consistency been shown to reduce length of stay and have lower blood loss, which is offset against its higher costs when compared to open surgery.

Radiotherapy

The current standard of care is intensity modulated radiotherapy (IMRT) with escalated dosing of 76–80 Gy and a period of ADT.

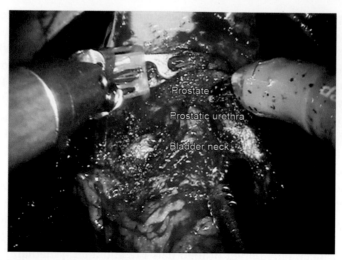

Fig. 11.2: Robotic radical prostatectomy—intraoperative image.

Bolla et al. published their RCT on EBRT versus EBRT and ADT in 2010. They randomised 415 with T3–T4 prostate cancer and found a 25% improvement in 10-year CSS in patients who received adjuvant ADT.[38]

Some felt that the ADT was having the primary effect rather than the radiotherapy. However, subsequently multiple studies have shown that the addition of radiotherapy to ADT does improve survival over ADT alone. The SPGC-7 study by Widmark et al. showed a 12% 10-year improvement in CSM with the addition of flutamide. With a median of 7.6-year follow-up bDFS was 82.4%.[21]

Another notable paper is the PRO7 trial where ADT was compared to ADT with IMRT and the combination treatment showed a 23% improvement in CSS after 6 years of follow-up.[39]

Currently, research is assessing the role of early or late radiotherapy in patients with T3 or high-risk disease or positive surgical margins after RRP, as up to 50% may develop local recurrence.[40] RADICALS is one such UK-based trial comparing salvage or immediate radiotherapy with or without hormonal manipulation.[41] Three other trials, which have published their data, are the SWOG 8794, EORTC 22911 and the ARO 96-02.[42-44] All have shown an improvement in bDFS with early radiotherapy but only the SWOG study showed an improvement in metastases free survival or overall survival (OS).

Brachytherapy

Brachytherapy for localised prostate cancer has been in use since the late 1980s and has shown similar results to EBRT with bDFS of between 71% and 96% at five-year follow-up.[45] It is classically delivered as low dose permanently implanted prostatic seeds (iodine-125 or palladium-103) or more recently as temporary high-dose seeds (HDR-Brachytherapy with iridium-192). HDR therapy is normally performed in high risk/T3 disease and is commonly given with a course of EBRT and ADT. Generally accepted patient selection criteria for low-dose brachytherapy include:

- Stage cT1b-T2a N0, M0
- Gleason score < 6
- PSA < 10 ng/mL
- <50% of biopsy cores involved with cancer
- Prostate volume of < 50 cm^3
- International Prostatic Symptom Score < 12

Potters et al. reported results for 1,449 consecutive patients having brachytherapy, with "high-risk" patients also receiving EBRT. Sixty-one per cent of patients had T1c disease and 33% had T2a disease. After 12 years of follow-up, the OS was 81% and CSS was 93%. In this series, bDFS appeared to be unaffected by either hormone use or the addition of EBRT.[46]

Minimally Invasive Treatments

Cryotherapy uses freezing treatments to induce cell death by dehydration, protein denaturation, ice crystal formation, which results in cellular rupture and vascular stasis, thrombi formation and ischaemia. It may also induce an immune response towards the cancerous cells. Whole gland therapy has a large evidence base and a series of 590 patients with 5.4 year mean follow-up, by Bahn et al in 2002, reported a bDFS of 92% for low-risk, 89% for intermediate-risk and 89% for high- risk cancer.[47] Similar results were reported by Rodriguez et al. on 108 patients with a median follow-up of five years. They showed a bDFS of 96.4% for low-risk, 91.2% for intermediate- risk and 62% for high-risk tumours.[48] An RCT comparing whole gland cryotherapy to EBRT also found no difference.[49] These outcomes compare favourably to studies assessing outcomes of primary focal cryotherapy which have reported a bDFS between 71% and 93% at follow-ups ranging from 9 months to 70 months.[50,51]

HIFU uses focused ultrasound waves to induce mechanical and thermal tissue damage along with cavitation, which results in coagulative necrosis. Crouzet et al. published a large single centre study of whole gland treatment in 1002 patients with T1 or T2 disease who were unsuitable for radical surgery. The eight-year bDFS for low-, intermediate- and high-risk disease patients were 76%, 63% and 57% respectively. The 10-year OS and CSS were 80% and 97% respectively.[52]

Side Effects

All the radical and whole gland treatments have a high level of morbidity particularly in terms of continence and erectile dysfunction (ED). The robotic technique for RRP has significantly reduced the early operative complications. Continence rates after RRP ranges between 69% and 92.5% whilst ED rates range from 10% to 50% at one year.

Assessing toxicity from radiotherapy using the modified Radiotherapy and Oncology Group scale (RTOG), 22.8% can develop grade 2 bowel, bladder and lymphatic complications and late grade 3–4 complications including death in < 5%.[53] Secondary malignancies of the rectum and bladder have also been reported. In addition, brachytherapy may result in the need for TURP in up to 9% of cases.

A meta-analysis showed one-year potency rates of 76% for brachytherapy, 60% for combined brachytherapy and EBRT, 55% for EBRT alone, 34% with a nerve sparing RRP and 25% for open RRP.[54]

Comparably, high side-effects also occur with whole gland cryotherapy and a Cochrane review by Shelly et al. in 2007 found impotence rates of 47–100%, incontinence in 1.3–19%, urethral sloughing in 3.9–85%, fistulae in 0–2%, bladder-neck obstruction in 2–55%, stricture in 2.2–17% and pain in 0.4–3.1%.[55]

Primary focal cryotherapy studies report a much better side-effect profile with incontinence rates of from 0% to 3.6% and ED in 0–42%. Haematuria, strictures and rectal fistulae are also very rare.

Improvements in the HIFU device have resulted in a decrease in incontinence from 6.4% to 3.1% and bladder outflow obstruction from 34.9% to 5.9%. Furthermore, only 0.4% of all patients developed rectourethral fistulae.

Key Points

- The most common treatment options are AS, radical treatments such as RRP, EBRT, brachytherapy or focal treatments such as cryotherapy or HIFU.
- All the radical and whole gland treatments have a high level of side effects particularly with regards to continence and ED.

METASTATIC DISEASE

Prostate cancer cells are under the influence of androgens, 90% of which are secreted by the testes and 10% by the adrenal glands. The hypothalamic–pituitary–gonadal axis controls their secretion. Luteinizing hormone secreting hormone (LHRH) from the hypothalamus stimulates the anterior pituitary to secrete luteinizing hormone (LH), which stimulates the Leydig cells of the testes to secrete testosterone.

Treatment of advanced and metastatic prostate cancer has largely been with hormonal manipulation/ADT by either blockade of the androgen receptor, by disrupting the hypothalamic–pituitary–gonadal axis (LHRH antagonists/agonists) or by preventing secretion with bilateral orchidectomy.

Surgical or chemical castration is the ultimate goal, where currently we aim for a testosterone level of <20 ng/mL (0.7 nmol/L).[56]

Recent data suggest that the drop to nadir PSA level after starting ADT is closely correlated with prognosis. The SWOG 9346 trial found that median survival for a patients with a nadir PSA after seven months of <0.2 ng/mL was 75 months, PSA of 0.2–4 ng/mL was 44 months and for a PSA > 4 ng/mL was 13 months.[57]

Others have also tried to identify poor prognostic groups such as with visceral metastases, high-grade disease, high-presenting PSA and high PSADT after reaching a nadir.

Patients on ADT develop side effects such as loss of libido, hot flushes, gynaecomastia, breast pain, osteoporosis, increased risk of diabetes and cardiovascular disease, which can limit their quality of life (QoL). Several trials assessing intermittent androgen therapy (IAT) have concluded that there is no detriment to OS and there may be some benefit in improving QoL. Thus, a well-informed patient may be treated with IAT until a state of castrate resistance develops.

After 18–24 months patients eventually develop a castrate resistance state where PSA continues to rise despite castrate testosterone levels. The current definition is three consecutive PSA rises, one week apart with 2 PSAs rising >50% over the nadir.

Classically, initial treatment has been the use of maximum androgen blockade with the addition of anti-androgens such as bicalutamide to the LHRH agonist. Once this fails a trial of anti-androgen withdrawal is normally performed, which can lead to a PSA response in up to 30%. Subsequently, in patients with a good performance status docetaxel was the chemotherapeutic agent of choice. The TAX 327 study showed a two-month survival advantage for patients having docetaxel + prednisolone versus mitoxantrone + prednisolone.[58]

Recently, although newer treatments such as abiraterone, enzalutamide and cabazitaxel have become available, which have been assessed in the pre- and post-docetaxel setting.

Abiraterone is a CYP17 inhibitor, which prevents intra-cellular testosterone synthesis and is usually administered alongside prednisolone. It gives approximately a median five-month survival advantage in both the pre- and postdocetaxal setting.[59-61]

Enzalutamide is a new anti-androgen, which blocks the androgen receptor and also prevents its translocation and transcription. The PREVAIL trial assessing enzalutamide in the predocetaxal setting was stopped after an interim analysis. After a median of 22-month follow-up an 81% relative reduction in radiographic progression free survival and a 29% relative risk reduction of death was seen in favour of enzalutamide. Previously, a median 5.8 month improved survival had been seen in the post-docetaxal setting.[62,63]

Cabazitaxel is a taxane derivative, which has been shown to have a median 2.4 month improved survival in the post-docetaxel setting.[64]

The exact sequence of these drugs remains to be determined and hopefully future research and ultimately availability of these compounds will determine their exact position in the treatments of metastatic castrate resistant prostate cancer.

Recent work has focused into chemoreduction and two large database studies have shown improved survival in patients who have had radical treatments.[65,66] Going into the future treating the local tumour in patients with metastatic disease may convey a survival benefit. Only well-designed RCTs will be able to answer this question.

REFERENCES

1. Schroder FH, Hugosson J, Roobol MJ, et al. Prostate-cancer mortality at 11 years of follow-up. The New England journal of medicine. 2012;366(11):981-90.
2. Kilpelainen TP, Tammela TL, Malila N, et al. Prostate cancer mortality in the Finnish randomized screening trial. Journal of the National Cancer Institute. 2013;105(10):719-25.
3. Hugosson J, Carlsson S, Aus G, et al. Mortality results from the Goteborg randomised population-based prostate-cancer screening trial. The Lancet Oncology. 2010;11(8):725-32.
4. Andriole GL, Crawford ED, Grubb RL, et al. Prostate cancer screening in the randomized Prostate, Lung, Colorectal, and Ovarian Cancer Screening Trial: mortality results after 13 years of follow-up. Journal of the National Cancer Institute. 2012;104(2):125-32.
5. Ilic D, Neuberger MM, Djulbegovic M, et al. Screening for prostate cancer. The Cochrane database of systematic reviews. 2013;1:CD004720.
6. Hossack T, Patel MI, Huo A, et al. Location and pathological characteristics of cancers in radical prostatectomy specimens identified by transperineal biopsy compared to transrectal biopsy. The Journal of urology. 2012;188(3):781-5.
7. Bott SR, Young MP, Kellett MJ, et al. Contributors to the UCLHTRPD. Anterior prostate cancer: is it more difficult to diagnose? BJU international. 2002;89(9): 886-9.
8. Nelson AW, Harvey RC, Parker RA, et al. Repeat prostate biopsy strategies after initial negative biopsy: meta-regression comparing cancer detection of transperineal, transrectal saturation and MRI guided biopsy. PloS one. 2013;8(2):e57480.
9. Loeb S, Vellekoop A, Ahmed HU, et al. Systematic review of complications of prostate biopsy. European urology. 2013;64(6):876-92.
10. Barzell WE, Melamed MR. Appropriate patient selection in the focal treatment of prostate cancer: the role of transperineal 3-dimensional pathologic mapping of the prostate—a 4-year experience. Urology. 2007;70(6 Suppl):27-35.
11. Onik G, Miessau M, Bostwick DG. Three-dimensional prostate mapping biopsy has a potentially significant impact on prostate cancer management. Journal of clinical oncology : official journal of the American Society of Clinical Oncology. 2009;27(26):4321-6.
12. Grey A, Chana M, Popert R, et al. The diagnostic accuracy of MRI PI-RADS scoring in a transperineal prostate biopsy setting. BJU international. 2014.

13. Puech P, Potiron E, Lemaitre L, et al. Dynamic contrast-enhanced-magnetic resonance imaging evaluation of intraprostatic prostate cancer: correlation with radical prostatectomy specimens. Urology. 2009;74(5):1094-9.
14. Haffner J, Lemaitre L, Puech P, et al. Role of magnetic resonance imaging before initial biopsy: comparison of magnetic resonance imaging-targeted and systematic biopsy for significant prostate cancer detection. BJU international. 2011;108(8 Pt 2):E171-8.
15. Siddiqui MM, Rais-Bahrami S, Truong H, et al. Magnetic resonance imaging/ultrasound-fusion biopsy significantly upgrades prostate cancer versus systematic 12-core transrectal ultrasound biopsy. European urology. 2013;64(5): 713-9.
16. Itatani R, Namimoto T, Atsuji S, et al. Negative predictive value of multiparametric MRI for prostate cancer detection: Outcome of 5-year follow-up in men with negative findings on initial MRI studies. European journal of radiology. 2014.
17. Abd-Alazeez M, Ahmed HU, Arya M, et al. The accuracy of multiparametric MRI in men with negative biopsy and elevated PSA level—can it rule out clinically significant prostate cancer? Urologic oncology. 2014;32(1):45 e17-22.
18. Thompson JE, Moses D, Shnier R, et al. Multiparametric Magnetic Resonance Imaging Guided Diagnostic Biopsy Detects Significant Prostate Cancer and could Reduce Unnecessary Biopsies and Over Detection: A Prospective Study. The Journal of urology. 2014.
19. Albertsen PC, Hanley JA, Fine J. 20-year outcomes following conservative management of clinically localized prostate cancer. JAMA : the journal of the American Medical Association. 2005;293(17):2095-101.
20. Bill-Axelson A, Holmberg L, Garmo H, et al. Radical prostatectomy or watchful waiting in early prostate cancer. The New England journal of medicine. 2014;370(10):932-42.
21. Widmark A, Klepp O, Solberg A, et al. Endocrine treatment, with or without radiotherapy, in locally advanced prostate cancer (SPCG-7/SFUO-3): an open randomised phase III trial. Lancet. 2009;373(9660):301-8.
22. Eggener SE, Scardino PT, Walsh PC, et al. Predicting 15-year prostate cancer specific mortality after radical prostatectomy. The Journal of urology. 2011;185 (3):869-75.
23. Ross HM, Kryvenko ON, Cowan JE, et al. Do adenocarcinomas of the prostate with Gleason score (GS) </=6 have the potential to metastasize to lymph nodes? The American journal of surgical pathology. 2012;36(9):1346-52.
24. Ahmed HU, Arya M, Freeman A, et al. Do low-grade and low-volume prostate cancers bear the hallmarks of malignancy? The Lancet Oncology. 2012;13(11): e509-17.
25. Lin D, Bayani J, Wang Y, et al. Development of metastatic and non-metastatic tumor lines from a patient's prostate cancer specimen-identification of a small subpopulation with metastatic potential in the primary tumor. The Prostate. 2010;70(15):1636-44.
26. Grasso CS, Wu YM, Robinson DR, et al. The mutational landscape of lethal castration-resistant prostate cancer. Nature. 2012;487(7406):239-43.
27. Bastian PJ, Mangold LA, Epstein JI, et al. Characteristics of insignificant clinical T1c prostate tumors. A contemporary analysis. Cancer. 2004;101(9):2001-5.
28. van As NJ, Norman AR, Thomas K, et al. Predicting the probability of deferred radical treatment for localised prostate cancer managed by active surveillance. European urology. 2008;54(6):1297-305.

29. Klotz L, Zhang L, Lam A, et al. Clinical results of long-term follow-up of a large, active surveillance cohort with localized prostate cancer. Journal of clinical oncology: official journal of the American Society of Clinical Oncology. 2010;28(1):126-31.

30. van den Bergh RC, Roemeling S, Roobol MJ, et al. Outcomes of men with screen-detected prostate cancer eligible for active surveillance who were managed expectantly. European urology. 2009;55(1):1-8.

31. Bill-Axelson A, Holmberg L, Ruutu M, et al. Radical prostatectomy versus watchful waiting in early prostate cancer. The New England journal of medicine. 2005;352(19):1977-84.

32. Bill-Axelson A, Holmberg L, Filen F, et al. Radical prostatectomy versus watchful waiting in localized prostate cancer: the Scandinavian prostate cancer group-4 randomized trial. Journal of the National Cancer Institute. 2008;100(16):1144-54.

33. Bill-Axelson A, Holmberg L, Ruutu M, et al. Radical prostatectomy versus watchful waiting in early prostate cancer. The New England journal of medicine. 2011;364(18):1708-17.

34. Wilt TJ, Brawer MK, Jones KM, et al. Radical prostatectomy versus observation for localized prostate cancer. The New England journal of medicine. 2012; 367(3):203-13.

35. Shikanov S, Song J, Royce C, et al. Length of positive surgical margin after radical prostatectomy as a predictor of biochemical recurrence. The Journal of urology. 2009;182(1):139-44.

36. Menon M, Bhandari M, Gupta N, et al. Biochemical recurrence following robot-assisted radical prostatectomy: analysis of 1384 patients with a median 5-year follow-up. European urology. 2010;58(6):838-46.

37. Engel JD, Kao WW, Williams SB, et al. Oncologic outcome of robot-assisted laparoscopic prostatectomy in the high-risk setting. Journal of endourology/ Endourological Society. 2010;24(12):1963-6.

38. Bolla M, Van Tienhoven G, Warde P, et al. External irradiation with or without long-term androgen suppression for prostate cancer with high metastatic risk: 10-year results of an EORTC randomised study. The Lancet Oncology. 2010;11 (11):1066-73.

39. Warde P, Mason M, Ding K, et al. Combined androgen deprivation therapy and radiation therapy for locally advanced prostate cancer: a randomised, phase 3 trial. Lancet. 2011;378(9809):2104-11.

40. Swanson GP, Thompson IM. Adjuvant radiotherapy for high-risk patients following radical prostatectomy. Urologic oncology. 2007;25(6):515-9.

41. Parker C, Sydes MR, Catton C, et al. Radiotherapy and androgen deprivation in combination after local surgery (RADICALS): a new Medical Research Council/ National Cancer Institute of Canada phase III trial of adjuvant treatment after radical prostatectomy. BJU international. 2007;99(6):1376-9.

42. Bolla M, van Poppel H, Tombal B, et al. Postoperative radiotherapy after radical prostatectomy for high-risk prostate cancer: long-term results of a randomised controlled trial (EORTC trial 22911). Lancet. 2012;380(9858):2018-27.

43. Wiegel T, Bartkowiak D, Bottke D, et al. Adjuvant Radiotherapy Versus Wait-and-See After Radical Prostatectomy: 10-year Follow-up of the ARO 96-02/AUO AP 09/95 Trial. European urology. 2014.

44. Thompson IM, Tangen CM, Paradelo J, et al. Adjuvant radiotherapy for pathological T3N0M0 prostate cancer significantly reduces risk of metastases and improves survival: long-term followup of a randomized clinical trial. The Journal of urology. 2009;181(3):956-62.

45. Peinemann F, Grouven U, Bartel C, et al. Permanent interstitial low-dose-rate brachytherapy for patients with localised prostate cancer: a systematic review of randomised and nonrandomised controlled clinical trials. European urology. 2011;60(5):881-93.

46. Potters L, Morgenstern C, Calugaru E, et al. 12-year outcomes following permanent prostate brachytherapy in patients with clinically localized prostate cancer. The Journal of urology. 2008;179(5 Suppl):S20-4.

47. Bahn DK, Lee F, Badalament R, et al. Targeted cryoablation of the prostate: 7-year outcomes in the primary treatment of prostate cancer. Urology. 2002;60 (2 Suppl 1):3-11.

48. Rodriguez SA, Arias Funez F, Bueno Bravo C, et al. Cryotherapy for primary treatment of prostate cancer: intermediate term results of a prospective study from a single institution. Prostate cancer. 2014;2014:571576.

49. Donnelly BJ, Saliken JC, Brasher PM, et al. A randomized trial of external beam radiotherapy versus cryoablation in patients with localized prostate cancer. Cancer. 2010;116(2):323-30.

50. Barqawi AB, Stoimenova D, Krughoff K, et al. Targeted focal therapy for the management of organ confined prostate cancer. The Journal of urology. 2014; 192(3):749-53.

51. Onik G, Vaughan D, Lotenfoe R, et al. "Male lumpectomy": focal therapy for prostate cancer using cryoablation. Urology. 2007;70(6 Suppl):16-21.

52. Crouzet S, Chapelon JY, Rouviere O, et al. Whole-gland ablation of localized prostate cancer with high-intensity focused ultrasound: oncologic outcomes and morbidity in 1002 patients. European urology. 2014;65(5):907-14.

53. Ataman F, Zurlo A, Artignan X, et al. Late toxicity following conventional radiotherapy for prostate cancer: analysis of the EORTC trial 22863. European journal of cancer. 2004;40(11):1674-81.

54. Robinson JW, Moritz S, Fung T. Meta-analysis of rates of erectile function after treatment of localized prostate carcinoma. International journal of radiation oncology, biology, physics. 2002;54(4):1063-8.

55. Shelley M, Wilt TJ, Coles B, et al. Cryotherapy for localised prostate cancer. The Cochrane database of systematic reviews. 2007(3):CD005010.

56. Oefelein MG, Feng A, Scolieri MJ, et al. Reassessment of the definition of castrate levels of testosterone: implications for clinical decision making. Urology. 2000;56(6):1021-4.

57. Hussain M, Tangen CM, Higano C, et al. Absolute prostate-specific antigen value after androgen deprivation is a strong independent predictor of survival in new metastatic prostate cancer: data from Southwest Oncology Group Trial 9346 (INT-0162). Journal of clinical oncology : official journal of the American Society of Clinical Oncology. 2006;24(24):3984-90.

58. Tannock IF, de Wit R, Berry WR, et al. Docetaxel plus prednisone or mitoxantrone plus prednisone for advanced prostate cancer. The New England journal of medicine. 2004;351(15):1502-12.

59. de Bono JS, Logothetis CJ, Molina A, et al. Abiraterone and increased survival in metastatic prostate cancer. The New England journal of medicine. 2011; 364(21):1995-2005.

60. Fizazi K, Scher HI, Molina A, et al. Abiraterone acetate for treatment of metastatic castration-resistant prostate cancer: final overall survival analysis of the COU-AA-301 randomised, double-blind, placebo-controlled phase 3 study. The Lancet Oncology. 2012;13(10):983-92.

61. Ryan CJ, Smith MR, de Bono JS, et al. Abiraterone in metastatic prostate cancer without previous chemotherapy. The New England journal of medicine. 2013;368(2):138-48.

62. Scher HI, Fizazi K, Saad F, et al. Increased survival with enzalutamide in prostate cancer after chemotherapy. The New England journal of medicine. 2012; 367(13):1187-97.

63. Beer TM, Armstrong AJ, Rathkopf DE, et al. Enzalutamide in metastatic prostate cancer before chemotherapy. The New England journal of medicine. 2014;371 (5):424-33.

64. de Bono JS, Oudard S, Ozguroglu M, et al. Prednisone plus cabazitaxel or mitoxantrone for metastatic castration-resistant prostate cancer progressing after docetaxel treatment: a randomised open-label trial. Lancet. 2010;376(9747): 1147-54.

65. Culp SH, Schellhammer PF, Williams MB. Might men diagnosed with metastatic prostate cancer benefit from definitive treatment of the primary tumor? A SEER-based study. European urology. 2014;65(6):1058-66.

66. Sooriakumaran P, Nyberg T, Akre O, et al. Comparative effectiveness of radical prostatectomy and radiotherapy in prostate cancer: observational study of mortality outcomes. Bmj. 2014;348:g1502.

12
Chapter

Phyllodes Tumour of Breast: Still a Challenge

Abhinav Arun Sonkar, Akshay Anand Agarwal,
Kul Ranjan Singh, Saumya Singh, Jitendra Kumar Kushwaha

INTRODUCTION

Johannes Muller first described a tumour of breast in 1838,[1] which was fleshy, contained cystic spaces, and had a leaf-like architecture. He coined the term cystosarcoma phyllodes[1] derived from Greek word *phullodes* meaning *leaf like*. Its malignant potential was first described by *Cooper and Ackerman* in 1943 and the disease was aptly renamed as phyllodes tumour (PT) by World Health Organization (WHO).[2] It is classified under a heterogenous group of "fibroepithelial tumours", which describes a spectrum of biphasic neoplasm comprising fibroadenoma (FA), PT, and breast hamartomas. These involve proliferation of both epithelial and stromal components. It accounts for <1% of all breast malignancies and <5% of soft tissue sarcomas[3] with a higher prevalence in American white and Asian population.[4] Triple assessment has standardized the diagnosis of the majority of breast lumps; however, in patients of PT, clinical, radiological and cytopathological examination in isolation or combination may not be of much help because of their poor accuracy.[5] Rarity of the disease, occasional difficulty in preoperative diagnosis, its tendency to recur and a poor response to chemotherapy and radiotherapy, all lead to a delay in diagnosis, difficulty in management and attendant morbidity.

CLINICAL PRESENTATION

The age at presentation of PT is variable with a median of 45 years, about two decades later than that of FA,[6] which is an important differential diagnosis. PT rarely afflict adolescent and younger females.[7] They usually present with a history of a unilateral long standing painless firm breast lump.[4] Rapid rate of growth and large size though suspicious for malignant PT are not so rare in benign and borderline PT. PT tend to be of smaller size in the western world[7] because of screening and earlier presentation. In the author's experience, PT are relatively large at presentation in developing countries, probably because of illiteracy, poverty and delay in diagnosis.

A classical case of PT is a female patient over 35 years presenting with a large irregular, rapidly growing lump usually in the upper and outer quadrant of breast[4] with shiny skin and dilated coursing veins. The skin over the lump may show a bluish discoloration whilst nipple retraction is uncom-mon, as is fixation to skin and pectoral muscles. Large tumours may present with ulceration. Twenty per cent of patients have palpable axillary lymph nodes but only 5% of these harbour metastases. There are occasional case reports of PT in males presenting with gynaecomastia, in association with FA.[8-10]

Key Points

- Large, unilateral, painless, rapidly progressing lump with bosselated surface.
- Median age of presentation is 45 years.
- Tumour fixation to skin and pectoral muscle is a rarity, as is nipple retraction.
- Axillary lymphadenopathy is present in 20%, but only 5% are malignant.

ROLE OF PREOPERATIVE INVESTIGATIONS

Imaging

High-resolution ultrasound (HRUSG) and mammography are often the first investigations to be performed.[5] However, none of the currently available radiological tools like HRUSG, mammography, contrast-enhanced com-puted tomography and magnetic resonance imaging (MRI) can discriminate PT from FA or differentiate benign from malignant PT with 100% accuracy.

High-Resolution Ultrasound

On HRUSG, PT is seen as a well circumscribed lesion with smooth walls and edges exhibiting low internal echoes.[11] They appear heterogeneous rep-resenting solid areas interspread with cystic fluid filled spaces along with septations and are usually devoid of microcalcifications. PTs usually have smaller ratio of length to anteroposterior diameter compared with FA[12] and exhibit good transmission devoid of posterior acoustic enhancement. Cystic areas within a solid lesion is a hallmark of PT.[11]

Mammography

Mammography does not provide any extra-information over and above HRUSG. PT has well-defined borders, at times lobulated with or without coarse micro-calcification, often difficult to differentiate from FA.[11,13-16] The only hallmark defined for PT on mammography is a zone of radiolucency around the lesion, which is due to the pressure effect of the tumour and represents itself as a halo.[13-16] However, the halo sign is a tell-tale sign of most benign pathologies of the breasts.[17]

Magnetic Resonance Imaging

The PT appears well circumscribed, lobulated lesions having intramural septations on MRI. The differentiating features include internal anatomical variation within the lesion, along with expression of time-signal intensity curve, which has a rapid pattern.

The MRI has shown its usefulness in the diagnosis of PT > 3 cm or when it is very close to the chest wall where other modalities fail.[15] In larger PTs (>3 cm) specific dynamic enhancement patterns indicating malignant nature are observed,[15] which include a characteristic leafy and lobulated pattern best picked up by a subtraction MRI. High signal intensity on T_2-weighted images corresponds to haemorrhage and cystic changes. Increased Vmax (systolic peak velocity), PI (pulsatility index) and RI (resistance index) also characterize PT.[16] Proton magnetic resonance spectroscopy,[19] positron emission tomography scan[18] and scintimammography[20,21] may be of help; however, these investigations are yet to find a place in standard imaging protocols for PT.

Role of Pathological Analysis

Macroscopically, PT varies from being small to large and PT >20 cm in diameter have been reported. Smaller PTs often resemble FAs in being solid, compact tumours of small size, grey in colour, lobulated and at times having a cystic consistency. Giant PTs (>10 cm) constitute about 20% of all PTs and often exhibit reddish grey, flesh like areas with unequal distribution of necrotic gelatinous and hemorrhagic areas. However, the size of PT is not predictive of malignant histotype.

Fine-Needle Aspiration Cytology

On cytopathology, PTs are characterised by a dimorphic distribution of stromal and epithelial elements. PT stroma is highly distinctive and contains cohesive stromal cells with well-marked borders. Nuclear atypia, isolated stromal cells with naked nuclei and hyperplasia of ductal cells without apocrine cells are often found. Dispersed stromal cells with spindle-like nuclei, if >30% of total cells are diagnostic of PT.[22] This hyperplasia and hypercellularity of stroma differentiates PT from FA. Epithelial clusters in PT although quiescent are >1 mm in size, undulating and elongated as opposed to flattened and blunt clusters seen in FA.[23] These epithelial elements found in benign PT are absent in malignant lesions.[24] Cellular pleomorphism, hypercellularity with nuclear hyperchromatism and aberrant mitoses are indicators of malignant PT.[25,26] Due to the heterogeneous nature of tumour morphology, it often suffers from sampling errors and close to a quarter of lesions remain undiagnosed.[27,28]

The preoperative diagnosis of PT continues to challenge pathologists and surgeons alike. The presence of more than two features of combined clinical, radiological and cytopathological findings incorporated into "Paddington clinicopathological suspicious score" mandates a core biopsy of the lesion (Table 12.1).[28]

Core Needle Biopsy

Core biopsy provides a large amount of tissue with all the components; therefore, its diagnostic accuracy compared with cytopathology is better. On histopathology, PT may lack a true capsule,[29] exhibiting a hypercellular stromal component with increased mitotic activity along with cystic spaces lined by an epithelial component in papillary protrusion-like fashion with exaggerated intra canalicular proliferation. This stromal proliferation is most abundant in periductal areas and is heterogeneous in nature compared with FA, where it is uniform without atypia or increased mitoses. Although core biopsy, suffers from sampling errors like cytopathology it is more useful as the yield of tissue is increased and the preoperative differentiation between benign and malignant PT may be possible.[28-32]

The criteria proposed by Azzopardi[29] and Salvadori et al.[32] is considered the gold standard in distinguishing benign from malignant PT based on stromal hypercellularity, cellular atypia, tumour margins (pushing or infiltrative), tumour necrosis and increased mitoses (Table 12.2).

Table 12.1: Criteria for preoperative biopsy.

Paddington clinicopathological suspicious score

Clinical findings:
- Sudden increase in size in a longstanding breast lesion.
- Apparent fibroadenoma >3 cm in diameter in a patient >35 years.

Imaging:
- Rounded borders with a lobulated appearance at mammography.
- Alternation of cystic areas within a solid mass on high-resolution ultrasound.

Cytopathologic findings:
- Presence of hyper cellular stromal fragments.
- Indeterminate features.

Table 12.2: Azzopardi and Salvadori criteria for diagnosis of nature of phyllodes tumour.

Criteria	Histological type		
	Benign	Borderline	Malignant
Tumour margins	Pushing	↔	Infiltrative
Stromal cellularity	Low	Moderate	High
Mitotic rate (per 10 hpf)	<5	5–9	>10
Pleomorphism	Mild	Moderate	Severe

Immunohistochemistry and Molecular Analysis

Flow-cytometric estimation of S-phase fraction/DNA ploidy, p53 expression and Ki67 index assist in histological grading and may be of help in predicting the clinical outcome. The expression of CD10 varies in various subtypes of fibroepithelial tumours of the breast with greater expression in PT compared to FA. Increased expression of CD 10 is associated with greater malignant and metastatic potential in PT.[33] Tse *et al.* also noted a positive correlation between nitric oxide synthase (NOS) expression in stromal cells and tumour grade along with vascular endothelium derived growth factor and micro-vessel density.[34] A high expression of stromal NOS correlates with malignancy, but its role is questionable in predicting malignant progression and potential to metastasize. Stromal endothelin 1 (ET 1) expression[35] correlates well with atypical histological features and may have a limited role in tumour recurrence. Recently, hypoxia inducible factor 1 alpha was proposed to help in predicting the grade of PT and its metastatic potential. Its over expression is said to reduce the disease free survival thus offering a platform for development of newer targeted therapies.[36]

Key Points

- Preoperative pathological analysis plays the most pivotal role in diagnosis of PT.
- Core needle biopsy has a distinct role.
- Role of IHC and molecular analysis is only supportive and not diagnostic.
- Criteria proposed by Azzopardi–Salvadori and Paddington clinico-pathological suspicious score gives better insight in preoperative diagnosis and stratification (Table 12.2).

Other recently explored molecules include ras homolog enriched in brain (RHEB), histone deacetylase 1(HDAC1) and WEE1homolog (WEE1).[37] RHEB has a role in cell growth and the cell cycle. HDAC1 determines the tumour progression and thus prognosis, whereas WEE1 belonging to nuclear kinase is a tumour suppressor. Both FA and PT express these proteins but their levels differ. Expression of RHEB and HDAC1 is highest in PT and determines tumourigenesis in the stromal component. The expression frequencies of RHEB, HDAC1 and WEE1 proteins were found to be highest in epithelial cells of normal breast tissue, intermediate in FA and lowest in PT. However, the usefulness of these molecules in diagnosis of PT is yet to be standardized.[37]

Prognostic Factors

The prognosis of PT is determined by various factors, histopathology being strongest of all. On histopathology, mitotic figures greater than three per high power field, stromal over growth with atypia, tumour necrosis, infiltrating margins, mixed mesenchymal components are all associated with poor prognosis. Multivariate analyses have shown that histological type and tumour necrosis seem to be most potent prognostic factors.[38] It is the borderline and malignant PT that most commonly metastasizes. Patients with metastasis and lymph node involvement have a poor prognosis and decreased survival.[39] P53 over-expression is a marker of poor prognosis, as is increased telomerase activity, which is detected by flow-cytometric analysis.

Most of the malignant tumours are large in size,[40] but no correlation exists between the recurrence and size of the primary lesion; however, size is an important predictor of metastasis. Age is not an independent factor but patients presenting in adolescence have a less aggressive course compared to their older counterparts.[16,17] After surgery, benign, borderline and malignant PT have five-year disease-free survival of 96%, 74% and 66%, respectively.[41]

Key Points

- Prognosis depends on histopathology and tumour margins after resection.
- Expression of molecular markers like p53, Ki67 and telomerase are being investigated.
- Five-year disease-free survival after surgery for benign, borderline and malignant disease is 96%, 74% and 66%, respectively.

MANAGEMENT

Surgery for Primary Lesion

Surgery forms the mainstay in the management of PT and ranges from wide local excision with a margin of normal breast tissue to mastectomy depending on the histological grade and clinical behaviour of the tumour.[42]

Unlike four decades ago, when radical surgery was standard treatment for all PTs without due consideration of histopathology or tumour size and behaviour, surgical management has become more conservative, based on the fact that radical surgery does not offer added survival advantage. Enucleation or shelling out of PT irrespective of histological type has been abandoned owing to a higher rate of recurrence.[42] Controversy exists regarding the extent of surgery especially for borderline and malignant PT. PT diagnosed preoperatively, must undergo a wide local excision with a margin of at least 1 cm all around the tumour, especially for borderline and malignant PT.

The PT irrespective of tumour histological grade, diagnosed after local excision should be closely followed whilst those with positive margin should undergo re-excision with a margin of 1 cm.[27,43] Wide local excision is an adequate procedure as long as the tumour to breast size permits, leading to breast conservation. If it is a giant (>10 cm) PT then mastectomy is preferred with intent to remove the entire visible tumour.

Clinically, palpable lymph nodes are present in 20% of all PTs, whereas histopathological evidence of metastasis is present in <5%.[42] The major route of metastasis is hematogenous. Lymph node involvement is a rarity and does not warrant routine axillary lymph node dissection until there is pathological evidence of metastatic deposits.[27,41,43] Norris and Taylor[31] have suggested that if lymph nodes are large enough one low lying lymph node should be taken for histopathological examination, a concept similar to sentinel lymph node in breast cancer. Sometimes, patients with giant PTs have multiple enlarged lymph nodes suspicious of malignancy. Should lymph nodes be found to be metastatic on frozen section, axillary lymph node dissection may be done. In the absence of frozen section, axillary lymph node dissection seems to be a safe bet. However, there is dearth of literature on this specific issue. A suggestive flowchart for management of PT is shown in Flowchart 12.1.

Breast Conserving Surgery and Reconstruction

Reconstruction offers emotional well-being with a better quality of life. Reconstruction of the breast does not interfere in the recognition of recurrent tumour.[44] Breast conserving surgery with wide local excision has recurrence rates similar to mastectomy if oncological principles are adhered to. Breast reconstruction can be performed immediately after primary surgery or after an interval. Breast reconstruction is done with pedicle flaps; transverse rectus abdominis myocutaneous and latissimus dorsi (LD) flap being commonly used. Breast prosthesis, such as tissue expanders/saline implants and Alloderm are used when subcutaneous tissue is scanty. In breast reconstruction surgery, the nipple areola complex (NAC) is often spared for better cosmetic results. Sparing NAC is controversial in centrally located tumours and may be sacrificed and reconstructed with skin grafts and tattooing. Good results are obtained when an LD flap with implants is used.[44] However, newer surgical techniques are needed to fulfil the growing need of reconstruction.

Key Points

- Wide local excision with a margin of >1 cm is standard treatment, irrespective of the nature of disease.
- In giant PT (>10 cm), mastectomy is preferred.
- Axillary lymph node dissection is not routinely warranted due to rarity of metastasis in the lymph node.
- Breast reconstruction should be considered in patients undergoing mastectomy. It offers better quality of life.

Flowchart 12.1: Management of phyllodes tumour.

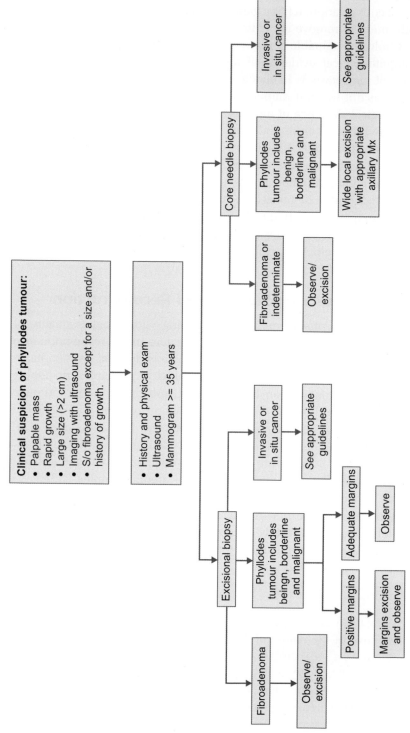

Recurrence and Metastasis: Factors and Guidelines for Treatment

Despite the best efforts of surgical management, PT has a tendency to recur locally and most commonly within the first few years following surgery. The rate of recurrence is maximum for borderline and malignant PT (30–65%) followed by benign PT (15–30%).[27,28,41,43,45,46] In the majority of cases recurrence presents as an isolated lesion resembling the original tumour albeit with increased cellularity and aggressive histological features. Positive margins after excision determine local recurrence. Recurrence of benign PT is managed with wide local excision whilst mastectomy is reserved for borderline or malignant PT. At times, aggressive widespread recurrence with chest wall and lung parenchyma involvement may necessitate active palliation with extended excision, reconstruction and radiotherapy (Flowchart 12.2).

Key Points

- Local recurrence is more common than distant metastasis, seen maximally in borderline and malignant PT.
- Distant metastasis occurs rarely, lungs followed by bone, heart and liver being common sites.
- Adjuvant radiotherapy can be considered in PT having recurrence with invasion to chest wall or inadequate margin.
- Role of chemotherapy and endocrine therapy has not well established.

Distant metastases occur in 10% of the patients with the lungs being most commonly involved followed by bone, heart, liver and abdominal viscera. If malignant PT metastasizes, it usually does so in the first 10 years of index surgery with or without local recurrence or involvement of lymph nodes.[27,28,41,43,45,46] Histopathological examination of metastatic disease shows aberrant stromal fragments, atypia, overgrowth, high mitotic index, tumour necrosis with no evidence of epithelial elements. The risk of metastasis is not determined by tumour margin positivity after initial surgery but by tumour behaviour and biology. Adjuvant radiotherapy is strongly favoured in PT with chest wall invasion or if the margins are <1 cm with inadequate resection.[47,48] Wide local excision of malignant and borderline PT with negative margins combined with adjuvant radiotherapy has led to a reduction of the recurrence rate from 86% to 59%.[48] Both radiotherapy and chemotherapy are not routinely indicated.[26,27,41,43] There is high epithelial expression of oestrogen receptor (58%) and progesterone receptor (75%), singly or in combination, and the level decreases with increasing degree of malignancy. Despite PT being oestrogen receptor, progesterone receptor positive, endocrine therapy and adjuvant cytotoxic chemotherapy have no proven role in treatment.[49] A flowchart for management of recurrent PT is given in Flowchart 12.2.

Flowchart 12.2: Management of recurrent and metastatic PT.

```
        ┌─────────────────────────────────┐
        │ Locally recurrent breast mass   │
        │ following excision of phyllodes │
        │ tumour                          │
        └─────────────────────────────────┘
                       │
        ┌─────────────────────────────────┐
        │ • History and physical exam     │
        │ • USG breast and axilla         │
        │ • Mammogram                     │
        │ • Tissue sampling               │
        │   (histology preferred)         │
        │ • Consider chest imaging        │
        └─────────────────────────────────┘
              │                       │
   ┌─────────────────────┐   ┌─────────────────────┐
   │ No metastatic       │   │ Metastatic disease  │
   │ disease             │   │                     │
   └─────────────────────┘   └─────────────────────┘
              │                       │
   ┌─────────────────────┐   ┌─────────────────────┐
   │ Re-excision with    │   │ Management following│
   │ wide margins with   │   │ principles of       │
   │ appropriate         │   │ soft tissue sarcoma │
   │ management of axilla│   └─────────────────────┘
   └─────────────────────┘
              │
   ┌─────────────────────┐
   │ Consider            │
   │ postoperative       │
   │ radiation           │
   └─────────────────────┘
```

CONCLUSION

Rarity of disease, comparative difficulty in preoperative histopathological diagnosis, propensity to recur and a poor response to chemotherapy and radiotherapy all lead to difficulty in management, delay in diagnosis of PT with attendant morbidity. Delay in presentation results in a large size making management more difficult. Histopathology remains the gold standard in making the diagnosis. Despite the best efforts at surgical management, PT has a tendency to recur locally and most commonly within the first few years of surgery. The size of the lesion has no bearing on recurrence. Radiotherapy finds favour in management of PT with chest wall invasion or if the margins are <1 cm with inadequate resection. Despite PT being oestrogen receptor, progesterone receptor positive, the role of endocrine and chemotherapy therapy has yet to be established.

Key Points

- A fibroepithelial tumour of breast.
- Accounts for <1% of all breast malignancy and <5% of soft tissue sarcoma.
- Mostly occurs between ages 40 and 50 years.
- Preoperative diagnosis is relatively difficult as many features mimic those of fibroadenoma.

- Surgery forms main stay of treatment, wide local excision with a margin of at least 1 cm should be applied irrespective of tumour behaviour.
- Chemotherapy, radiotherapy and hormonal manipulations have no proven role.
- PTs are notoriously known to recur locally whilst distant metastasis is uncommon.
- Breast reconstruction should be offered to patients postoperatively.

REFERENCES

1. Müller J. Uber den feineren Ban und Die Formen der Krankaften Geschwulste, vol. 1. Berlin: G Reiner;1838. pp.:54-7.
2. The World Health Organization. Histological typing of breast tumors—Second Edition. The World Organization. Am J Clin Pathol. 1982;78(6):806-16.
3. Dyer NH, Bridger JE, Taylor RS. Cystosarcoma phyllodes. Br J Surg. 1966;53(5): 450-5.
4. Bernstein L, Deapen D, Ross RK. The descriptive epidemiology of malignant cystosarcoma phyllodes tumours of the breast. Cancer. 1993;71(10):3020-4.
5. Umpleby HC, Moore I, Royle GT, et al. An evaluation of the preoperative diagnosis and management of cystosarcoma phyllodes. Ann R Coll Surg Engl. 1989;71(5):285-8.
6. Oberman HA. Cystosarcoma phyllodes; a clinicopathologic study of hypercel-lularperiductal stromal neoplasms of breast. Cancer. 1965;18:697-710.
7. Adachi Y, Matsushima T , Kido A, et al. Phyllodestumours in adolescents report of two cases and review of literature. Breast Dis. 1993;6:285-93.
8. West TL, Weiland LH, Clagett OT. Cystosarcoma phyllodes. Ann Surg. 1971; 173(4):520-8.
9. Pantoja E, Llobet RE, Lopez E. Gigantic cystosarcoma phyllodes in a man with gynecomastia. Arch Surg. 1976;111(5):611.
10. Reingold IM, Ascher GS. Cystosarcoma phyllodes in a man with gynaecomastia. Am J Clin Pathol. 1970;53(6):852-6.
11. Liberman L, Bonaccio E, Hamele-Bena D, et al. Benign and malignant phyl-lodes tumour: mammographic and sonographic findings. Radiology. 1996;198 (1):121-4.
12. Chao TC, Lo YF, Chen SC, et al. Sonographic features of phyllodes tumours of the breast. Ultrasound Obstet Gynecol. 2002;20(1):64-71.
13. Jorge Blanco A, Vargas Serrano B, Rodríguez Romero R, et al. Phyllodes tumours of the breast. Eur Radiol. 1999;9(2):356-60.
14. Cesmacini P, Zurrida S, Verohesi P, et al. Ultrasound, X-ray mammography and histopathology of cystosarcoma phyllodes. Radiology. 1983;146:1214.
15. Kinoshita T, Fukutomi T, Kubochi K. Magnetic resonance imaging of benign phyllodes tumours of the breast. Breast J. 2004;10(3):232-6.
16. Chao TC, Lo YF, Chen SC, et al. Phyllodes tumours of the breast. Eur Radiol. 2003;13(1):88-93.
17. Cosmacini P, Veronesi P, Zurrida S, et al. Mammography in the diagnosis of phyllodes tumours of the breast analysis of 99 cases. Radiol Med. 1991;82 (1-2):52-5.
18. Bakheet SM, Powe J, Ezzat A, et al. F-18 FDG whole-body positron emission tomography scan in primary breast sarcoma. Clin Nucl Med. 1998;23(9):604-8.

19. Tse GM, Cheung HS, Pang LM, et al. Characterization of lesions of the breast with proton MR spectroscopy: comparison of carcinomas, benign lesions, and phyllodes tumors. AJR Am J Roentgenol. 2003; 181(5):1267-72.

20. Katayama N, Inoue Y, Ichikawa T, et al. Increased activity in benign phyllodes tumour on Tc-99m MDP. Scintimammography. Clin Nucl Med. 2000;25(7): 551-2.

21. Ohta H, Komibuchi T, Nishio T, et al. Technetium-99m-sestamibi scinti-mammography of benign and malignant phyllodes tumours. Ann Nucl Med. 1997;11(1):37-9.

22. Krishnamurthy S, Ashfaq R, Shin HJ, et al. Distinction of phyllodes tumours from fibroadenoma a reappraisal of an old problem. Cancer. 2000;90(6):342-9.

23. Shimizu K, Korematsu M. Phyllodes tumor of the breast. A cytomorphologic approach based on evaluation of epithelial cluster architecture. Acta Cytol. 2002;46(2):332-6.

24. Blichert-Toft M, Hansen JP, Hansen OH, et al. Clinical course of cystosarcoma phyllodes related to histologic appearance. Surg Gynecol Obstet. 1975;140(6): 929-32.

25. Veneti S, Manek S. Benign phyllodes tumours vs. fibroadenoma: FNA cytologi-cal differentiation. Cytopathology. 2001;12(5):321-8.

26. Chen WH, Cheng SP, Tzen CY, et al. Surgical treatment of phyllodes tumours of the breast. Retrospective review of 172 cases. J Surg Oncol. 2005;91(3):185-94.

27. Ben Hassouna J, Damak T, Gamoudi A, et al. Phyllodes tumours of the breast: a case series of 106 patients. Am J Surg. 2006;192(2):141-7.

28. Jacklin RK, Ridgway PF, Ziprin P, et al. Optimizing preoperative diagnosis in phyllodes tumour of the breast. J Clin Pathol. 2006;59(5):454-9.

29. Azzopardi JG. Sarcoma of the breast. In: Bennigton J (Ed). Problems in Breast pathology Vol II, Major Problems in Pathology. Philadelphia, PA: WB Saunders; 1979. pp. 355-9.

30. Komenaka IK, El-Tamer M, Pile-Spellman E, et al. Core needle biopsy as a diag-nostic tool to differentiate phyllodes tumour from fibroadenoma. Arch Surg. 2003;138(9):987-90.

31. Norris HJ, Taylor HB. Relationship of histologic features to behavior of cysto-sarcoma phyllodes. Analysis of ninety-four cases. Cancer. 1967;20(12):2090-9.

32. Salvadori B, Cusumano F, Del Bo R, et al. Surgical treatment of phyllodes tumours of the breast. Cancer. 1989;63(12):2532-6.

33. Tse GM, Tsang AK, Putti TC, et al. Stromal CD10 expression in mammary fibro-adenomas and phyllodes tumours. J Clin Pathol. 2005;58(2):185-9.

34. Tse GM, Wong FC, Tsang AK, et al. Stromal nitric oxide synthase (NOS) expres-sion correlates with the grade of mammary phyllodes tumour. J Clin Pathol. 2005;58(6):600-4.

35. Tse GM, Chaiwun B, Lau KM, et al. Endothelin-1 expression correlates with atypical histological features in mammary phyllodes tumours. J Clin Pathol. 2007;60(9):1051-6.

36. Kuijper Al, van der Groep P, van der Wall E, et al. Expression of hypoxia-induc-ible factor 1 alpha and its downstream targets in fibroepithelial tumors of the breast. Breast Cancer Res. 2005;7(5):R808-18.

37. Eom M, Han A, Lee MJ, et al. Expressional difference of RHEB, HDAC1, and WEE1 proteins in the stromal tumours of the breast and their significance in tumour igenesis. Korean J Pathol. 2012;46(4):324-30.

38. Reinfuss M, Mituś J, Duda K, et al. The Treatment and prognosis of patients with phyllodes tumours of the breast. Cancer. 1996; 77(5):910-6.
39. Cohn-Cedermark G, Rutqvist LE, Rosendahl I, et al. Prognostic factors in cystosarcomaphyllodes. A clinicopathologic study of 77 patients. Cancer. 1991;68 (9):2017-22.
40. Vorherr H, Vorherr UF, Kutvirt DM, et al. Cystosarcoma phyllodes: epidemiology, pathohistology, pathobiology, diagnosis, therapy, and survival. Arch Gynecol. 1985;236(3):173-81.
41. Parker SJ, Harries SA. Phyllodes tumours. Postgrad Med J. 2001;77(909):428-35.
42. Liang MI, Ramaswamy B, Patterson CC, et al. Giant breast tumors: surgical management of phyllodes tumors, potential for reconstructive surgery and a review of literature. World J Surg Oncol. 2008;6:117.
43. Pandey M, Mathew A, Kattoor J, et al. Malignant phyllodes tumour. Breast J. 2001;7(6):411-6.
44. Crenshaw SA, Roller MD, Chapman JK. Immediate breast reconstruction with a saline implant and Alloderm, following removal of a Phyllodes tumour. World J Surg Oncol. 2011;9:34.
45. Cohn-Cedermark G, Rutqvist LE, Rosendahl I, et al. Prognostic factors in cystosarcoma phyllodes. A clinicopathological study of 77 patients. Cancer. 1991; 68(9):2017-22.
46. Norris HJ, Taylor HB. Relationship of histologic features to behavior of cystosarcoma phyllodes, analysis of ninety-four cases. Cancer. 1967;20(12):2090-9.
47. Soumarová R, Seneklová Z, Horová H, et al. Retrospective analysis of 25 women with malignant cystosarcoma phyllodes-treatment results. Arch Gynecol Obstet. 2004;269(4):278-81.
48. Barth RJ Jr, Wells WA, Mitchell SE, et al. A prospective multi-institutional study of adjuvant radiotherapy after resection of malignant phyllodes tumours. Ann Surg Oncol. 2009;16(8):2288-94.
49. Tse GM, Lee CS, Kung FY, et al. Hormonal receptors expression in epithelial cells of mammary phyllodes tumours correlates with pathologic grade of the tumour: a multicenter study of 143 cases. Am J Clin Pathol. 2002;118(4):522-6.

13

Chapter

Management of Patients with Primary Colorectal Cancer and Synchronous Liver Metastasis

Alistair AP Slesser, Elizabeth Smyth,
David Cunningham, Satvinder Mudan

INTRODUCTION

Approximately 40% of patients treated for colorectal cancer will develop liver metastases during their life time following treatment of the primary cancer, and these are defined as "metachronous" metastases. Approximately 15% of all patients diagnosed with colorectal cancer will have radiological evidence of liver metastases at the time of initial presentation,[1] and these are termed synchronous colorectal liver metastases (SCLM). It is the management of this group of patients which we will discuss. SCLM are accepted as indicative of a poor prognosis compared with metachronous lesions, consistently demonstrating more aggressive biological traits such as increased incidence of multiple, bilobar, large dimensional disease and thus irresectability.[2]

Colorectal liver metastases presenting within one year of the primary colorectal cancer are likely to behave biologically as those identified at the initial diagnosis, and this group of patients too will have an adverse biological behaviour from those who develop liver metastases several years later.[3]

Despite these apparent biological differences, the surgical management for both synchronous and metachronous liver metastases has, hitherto, been similar. The classical surgical strategy has been a sequential resection, whereby the primary tumour is resected first with subsequent adjuvant systemic chemotherapy followed by liver resection. Some centres are now undertaking a "reverse sequential" or "liver-first" approach, whereby the hepatic resection is performed first followed by the primary tumour resection for SCLM patients with rectal cancers on the postulate that in advanced rectal cancer the reverse strategy has a survival benefit, in sequential resections, by removing the main indicator of poor prognosis first thereby avoiding unnecessary rectal surgery in patients with incurable metastatic disease.[4,5] We consider the evidence supporting the different surgical approaches and impart our experience in managing this group of patients through the prism of a multidisciplinary team comprising academic surgeons, oncologists and radiologists in the institutional setting of an international comprehensive cancer centre.

Key Points

- Approximately 15% of all patients presenting with colorectal cancer will have liver metastases at the time of initial diagnosis, and at least 40% of the remainder of patients will go on to develop liver metastases at some time later.
- Synchronous colorectal liver metastases are an indicator of poor prognosis when compared with metachronous colorectal liver metastases and so likely represent a different biological group.
- Patients developing liver metastases within one year of diagnosis also demonstrate an adverse tumour biology similar to that of SCLM patients.

SELECTION FOR SURGERY

Full characterisation of the extent and distribution of disease is essential.[6,7] We recommend, all patients considered for radical treatment are evaluated by computed tomography (CT) of the chest, abdomen and pelvis, dedicated gadoxetic acid enhanced and diffusion-weighted magnetic resonance imaging (MRI) of the liver and 18F-FDG PET/CT to identify extra-hepatic metastases. Postchemotherapy morphological and functional metabolic response data[8-10] are used to aid in case selection. In the case of a rectal primary, pelvic MRI is performed.[11] All patients are discussed by the multidisciplinary team (MDT) in dedicated tumour-specific MDMs, where all relevant medical and ancillary disciplines are represented (Flowchart 13.1).

Untreated, patients with SCLM have an overall five-year survival of 3%.[1] Only surgical intervention offers possibility of long-term cure, and survival for patients rendered free of all evaluable disease ranges from 37% to 58%.[12] Previously held criteria for inoperability with a curative intent such as more than three liver lesions, bilobar distribution or extra-hepatic disease are no longer considered contraindications to a hepatic resection, provided all sites of disease can be adequately treated. We acknowledge that there is a growing interest towards complete resection in the presence of controllable serosal disease, retroperitoneal nodal disease and even for maximally debulking operations, and that debulking operations and that by these criteria between 15–13% of patients with SCLM will be found to be eligible for resection with a curative intent.[13]

In an era of effective chemotherapy, we consider that patients in whom all sites of disease can be controlled are potentially operable and our criteria for resectability in the liver is the ability to gain negative resection margins whilst leaving sufficient residual functional liver volume with adequate inflow and outflow to support the patient in the postoperative phase. The use of portal venous embolisation, downsizing chemotherapy, radiofrequency ablation and two-stage hepatectomies has increased the proportion of eligible patients.[14]

Flowchart 13.1: Algorithm for management of colorectal cancer patient presenting with synchronous liver metastases.

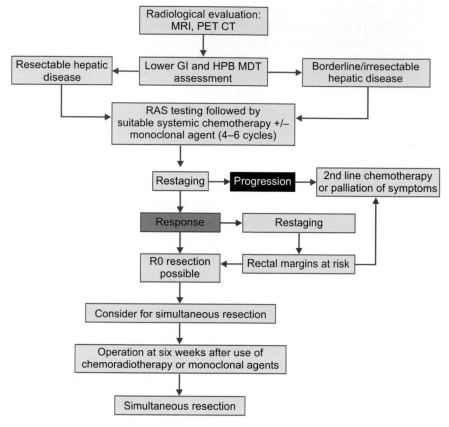

As the majority of the patients will have significant medical comorbidities, which will impact on the decision, timing and strategy for operation, close cooperation between the colorectal, hepatobiliary, anaesthetic and postoperative care teams is essential.[15]

Key Points

- Liver metastases are best characterised by MRI and extra-hepatic disease identified with 18-FDG CT/PET.
- All patients should be discussed by colorectal and hepatobiliary MDTs, and close cooperation is essential.
- SCLM is a signal of poor tumour biology and prognosis and should be considered for neoadjuvant chemotherapy to assess response, demonstrate the tumour biology and treat occult micrometastatic disease.
- The response to neoadjuvant systemic chemotherapy is an indicator of long-term oncological outcome and can be demonstrated by morphologic and functional imaging.

- Complete elimination of all evaluable disease remains the only chance of cure.
- Only approximately 15% of patients with synchronous colorectal liver metastases will have resectable liver disease at presentation, but the use of techniques such as portal vein embolisation and multimodal liver-directed therapies such as RFA and conversion systemic or regional chemotherapy can enlarge the pool of resectable patients by approximately 10%.
- Main determinant of whether a patient is a surgical candidate is the ability to control all sites of intra- and extra-hepatic disease and retain sufficient functional liver volume, usually 25% in good quality liver and 40% in damaged liver.

ONCOLOGICAL MANAGEMENT

The adverse prognosis of patients with SCLM is understood. At diagnosis the patient may have upfront resectable disease or borderline/irresectable metastases. For patients with de novo resectable disease, the EORTC 40983 trial, which randomised 364 operable patients to 12 cycles of perioperative FOLFOX (oxaliplatin plus fluorouracil) chemotherapy or surgery alone, demonstrated a three-year progression-free survival (PFS) benefit of 8.1% in favour of chemotherapy Hazrd Ratio = 0.77, range 0.60–1.00; $p = 0.041$.[16] This trial was underpowered for overall survival (OS) and revealed a non-statistically significant six-year OS benefit of 4.1% for patients treated with perioperative chemotherapy. A small proportion of patients (7% in EORTC 40983) progressed during chemotherapy, and these patients demonstrated an aggressive disease biology unlikely to benefit from resection and we consider such patients as inoperable for treatment with curative intent.

For a patient with borderline/irresectable disease receiving preoperative chemotherapy, the speed and quality of response as measured by dimensional, morphological and functional changes bear strongly correlated to a probability of eventual resection and to both PFS and OS.[17-19] This implies that the most appropriate active regimen should be selected, with the caveat that for most patients this will be part of a continuum of care due to the metastatic nature of the cancer. Doublet or triplet chemotherapy using a fluoropyrimidine backbone with the addition of either or both of irinotecan and oxaliplatin has been examined for the purpose of "conversion" to resectability; triplet combinations are not only associated with increased response rates but also with increased toxicity.[19,20]

The use of anti-angiogenic and anti-EGFR monoclonal antibodies (bevacizumab and cetuximab or panitumumab, respectively) has led to significant improvements in survival for patients with stage IV irresectable colorectal cancer, and these drugs may also improve outcomes for patients with resectable disease. However, it should be noted that most data are derived from trials that are not liver surgery specific, and consequently the absolute number of patients resected in any study is small, leading to significant inter-study heterogeneity and difficulty interpreting outcomes. Bevacizumab does not consistently increase response rates when added to cytotoxic chemotherapy, and this inconsistency is also reflected in liver resection rates in randomised trials. Although resection rates were increased from 6.4% to 8.1% in bevacizumab-treated patients in the NO16966 trial (Ox5FU ± bev), they were not significantly increased in other studies.[21,22] Despite these conflicting results, cytotoxic chemotherapy and bevacizumab for patients with RAS mutant SCLM remain a reasonable option as there is clear evidence that OS is improved.[23]

With respect to anti-EGFR therapy, extension of exon 2, 3 and 4 of *KRAS* and *NRAS* has aided in further refining the patient population who may benefit from these agents.[24] Retrospective analysis of chemotherapy plus cetuximab/panitumumab trials excluding patients with previously unexamined RAS mutations demonstrates that the addition of anti-EGFR therapy significantly increases response rates for these patients, independent of the chemotherapy companion arm.[24-26] For this reason, full RAS testing is recommended for all patients prior to initiation of anti-EGFR therapy. Increasingly, systemic therapy will become "personalised", maximising the therapeutic index and utilising cytotoxic and targeted biological agents.[27,28]

Key Points

- EORTC 40983 demonstrated that perioperative FOLFOX resulted in a three-year PFS benefit of 8.1% in patients with resectable disease.
- Patients may have "upfront" resectable metastases or borderline/irresectable disease. Response to preoperative chemotherapy correlates with conversion to resectability and also to OS.
- Although there is conflicting data, the use of bevacizumab is recommended in patients with RAS mutant as OS is shown to be improved.
- Extended RAS testing is necessary before considering anti-EGFR therapy.

OPERATIVE PLANNING

It is important to carefully consider both the effect of pre-existing liver damage, such as alcoholic or non-alcoholic steatohepatitis, and systemic chemotherapy on the functional and regenerative capacity of the remnant liver.[29] Most patients will have received at least doublet chemotherapy and likely, in addition, monoclonal agents such as bevacizumab. Irinotecan can induce steatohepatitis, fibrosis or even cirrhosis, and oxaliplatin may lead to sinusoidal injury and intra-hepatic veno-occlusive disease.[29] Preoperative, percutaneous biopsy of the future remnant liver should be considered in cases of concern. We believe an interval of 4 weeks before operation to be safe in the absence of VEGF inhibitors and 6 weeks if the latter agents have been deployed.[23]

We routinely only perform hepatic resections for patients with SCLM with a curative intent and a simultaneous resection where possible. In simultaneous resections, it is our preference for the colorectal primary to be resected first, by open operation and laparoscopically for a rectal primary. It is important in simultaneous resections that the anaesthetic delivery, surgical techniques and postoperative care are carefully considered, and if there are concerns during the colorectal phase such as unexpected complexity, blood loss or physiological performance then dialogue between the surgical teams may lead to deferment of the liver phase.[15]

Laparoscopic liver resection is uncommonly feasible as most patients have extensive liver disease requiring major hepatectomies. Intraoperative ultrasound is routinely used to confirm the location, size and anatomic relationship of metastases. Where the surgical field cannot encompass all sites of disease, for example bilobar disease, preoperative, intraoperative or postoperative radiofrequency ablation can be considered but with awareness of the limitations of RFA determined by proximity to intra-hepatic vascular structures and tumour size resulting in higher local recurrence rates up to 50% for lesions > 3 cm.[30] The development of microwave ablation therapy should increase the range of lesions treatable by such in situ ablative techniques.[31]

To avoid ischaemia on the chemotherapy-exposed liver, we do not use inflow clamping (Pringle manoeuvre). The Aquamantys System (Medtronic; Minneapolis, MN) bipolar coagulator prior to division with a cavitation ultrasonic aspirator (Valley Boulder, CO) is preferred for parenchymal transaction.[32] To avoid imaging artefact on follow-up MRI, we do not use any metal clips on the resection surface.

Key Points

- Low threshold to exclude chemotherapy-induced hepatic damage before proceeding with surgery.
- Primary tumour should be resected first during a simultaneous resection to allow the hepatic resection to be postponed if there are concerns regarding duration of surgery or blood loss.
- Anaesthetic techniques including low central venous pressure and oesophageal Doppler should be used to minimise the risks of surgery.
- Avoid metal clips to prevent future imaging artefact during follow-up.

DISCUSSION

The standard surgical treatment for patients with SCLM has been a sequential resection. Recently, however, there has been a growing trend to favour simultaneous resections in many centres.[33] There remain concerns about the safety and the long-term outcomes of simultaneous resections. This has led to most surgical units undertaking "simultaneous" resections in only a highly selected group of patients and restricted to straightforward colonic and hepatic resections.[33] Moreover, sequential resections tend to be favoured in patients considered to be high risk, that is the elderly, or patients with chemotherapy-induced hepatic damage requiring a substantial liver resection.[34] In a recent meta-analysis, we demonstrated that most centres had elected to perform sequential resections in patients with more extensive metastatic disease.[35] Where the patient's performance status is the source of concern, simultaneous resections may be inappropriate. We have demonstrated that, where the appropriate expertise exists, neither the extent of the metastatic burden nor the stage or location of the primary tumour should necessarily preclude simultaneous resections.[34]

Whether simultaneous resections for patients with SCLM have an oncological benefit when compared with sequential resections remains unclear, and the heterogeneity of disease burdens when comparing the two surgical strategies make reported data difficult to interpret.[35] Supporters of sequential resections feel that an interval prior to the hepatic resection permits progressive metastatic disease to declare itself and excludes such patients from further surgery and have concerns that simultaneous resections may leave behind occult micro-metastases in the remnant liver.[29,36] Analysis of our series of patients with SCLM undergoing simultaneous resections demonstrated that when stratified for extent of metastatic disease, those patients undergoing synchronous resections attained similar three-year overall and disease-free survivals to those treated by sequential resection.[34] In addition, it is thought that a better oncological result can be achieved with simultaneous resections by avoidance of the postoperative suppression of cell-mediated and humoral immunity and induction of pro-inflammatory and coagulopathic cascades as a consequence of firstly operation to resect the primary,[37-39] and then again at liver resection and moreover by avoiding the inevitably longer delay in the commencement of adjuvant chemotherapy associated with sequential resections.[40] A clear benefit of simultaneous resection is a reduction in the length of hospital stay by obviating the need for two admissions.[34,35]

The majority of studies comparing sequential versus simultaneous resections have a higher proportion of colonic primaries in the simultaneous resection group.[33,41] Rectal cancer resections and major hepatectomies dominate in our cohort of simultaneous resection for SCLM, and we have shown good postoperative and oncological outcomes.[34] Patient safety is key to selection regarding whether patients should undergo a sequential or a simultaneous resection. It is clear that a sequential approach will remain an important tool in the surgeon's armamentarium, particularly in patients where there are concerns regarding age or fitness or when an emergency primary tumour resection is required. Simultaneous resections are extensive and complex operations that should only be undertaken in centres where these procedures are routine. Moreover, it is essential that there is a close cooperation with all members of the multidisciplinary team, in particular a close association between the colorectal and liver surgical teams.[15]

Key Points

- Simultaneous resections are an emerging strategy for patients with SCLM.
- Sequential resections have a role when there are concerns regarding patient fitness, age or in an emergency presentation.
- Simultaneous resections prevent a delay in systemic chemotherapy and avoid the effect of postoperative immunosuppression associated with a sequential approach.
- Where the appropriate expertise exists, simultaneous resections are safe even for patients with rectal cancer or need for major liver resections.
- Simultaneous resections should only be undertaken in centres where they are routinely performed.

IRRESECTABLE SYNCHRONOUS COLORECTAL LIVER METASTASES

The majority of patients presenting with colorectal liver metastases will be initially found to have irresectable disease.[29] It is currently advised that all patients should receive neoadjuvant systemic chemotherapy.[29] Moreover, this strategy, if downsizing is sufficient, can render the metastatic disease resectable in between 12% and 40% of patients with initially irresectable disease,[42] and the use of monoclonal agents has been shown to increase this percentage.[21-27,43] With this approach, 5-year OS rates of 33% have been reported, almost replicating the OS rates of patients with initially resectable colorectal liver metastases.[42,43]

There is no consensus regarding the optimal management of the primary tumour in patients with irresectable liver disease. Management of the primary tumour should take into consideration the nature and severity of symptoms from the primary tumour and patient's wishes and comorbidities.[44,45] The treatment should aim to maintain or improve the patient's quality of life, control symptoms and prolong OS.[44,45] Patients with rectal cancer and who are capable of tolerating a major surgical intervention should be considered for chemoradiation when there is a high risk of obstruction or likelihood of developing debilitating pelvic symptoms. Otherwise, the following options should be considered: defunctioning colostomy, primary tumour resection, stenting, chemotherapy/chemoradiation or laser recanalisation to achieve effective palliation and equivalent survival.[46]

ADJUNCTIVE TREATMENTS

There is evidence to suggest that hepatic arterial infusion with chemotherapy combined with systemic chemotherapy, or intra-arterial infusion of yttrium-90 microspheres combined with systemic chemotherapy, show good response rates in patients with irresectable liver disease. However, despite improvements in time to progression, it remains unclear whether there is a translation into improved OS.[14,47]

The development of stereotactic body radiotherapy (SBRT) has been shown to have a low toxicity and can prevent progression in patients with limited hepatic disease and is now thought that SBRT will be a useful adjunct in the presence of limited irresectable disease.[14,47,48]

Key Points

- Majority of patients with SCLM will have irresectable disease on presentation.
- 12–40% of patients with intially irresectable disease can be converted to resectable disease with systemic chemotherapy.
- All patients with irresectable disease who can tolerate systemic chemotherapy should be so treated.
- Management of the colorectal primary should be according to whether it is symptomatic or asymptomatic. There are no clear guidelines on management, and it should be dictated by the patient's prognosis and wishes.
- Adjunctive therapies such as RFA and microwave ablation have a role to play particularly in irresectable disease. The use of RFA can increase the proportion of curative resections. SBRT is emerging as a useful adjunct in patients with irresectable limited hepatic disease.

EXTRA-HEPATIC METASTASES

Patients presenting with colorectal liver metastases and synchronous extra-hepatic disease pose a dilemma to both surgeons and oncologists. Until recently, the presence of extra-hepatic disease was considered an absolute contraindication to surgery. However, good five-year survival data of 28–40% are reported in patients, where the extra-hepatic disease is controlled by systemic or surgical treatment.[49]

Key Point

- The presence of extra-hepatic metastases is no longer an absolute contraindication to potentially curative liver resection in a highly selected group of patients.

FOLLOW-UP

Despite the many oncological and surgical advances in the management of patients with SCLM, the majority of patients will develop hepatic recurrence within two years following surgery with a curative intent. Close surveillance of patient's postcurative resection is essential as a significant proportion of patients who develop a hepatic recurrence will be amenable for further surgery.[29,50]

Key Point

- Close follow-up following curative hepatic resections is essential as the majority of patients will develop a recurrence, which will be amenable to further surgery.

REFERENCES

1. Manfredi S, Lepage C, Hatem C, et al. Epidemiology and management of liver metastases from colorectal cancer. Ann Surg. 2006;244(2):254-9.
2. Mantke R, Schmidt U, Wolff S, et al. Incidence of synchronous liver metastases in patients with colorectal cancer in relationship to clinico-pathologic characteristics. Results of a German prospective multicentre observational study. Eur J Surg Oncol. 2012;38(3):259-65. doi: 10.1016/j.ejso.2011.12.013.
3. Tsai MS, Su YH, Ho MC, et al. Clinicopathological features and prognosis in resectable synchronous and metachronous colorectal liver metastasis. Ann Surg Oncol. 2007;14(2):786-94.
4. Ayez N, Burger JW, van der Pool AE, et al. Long-term results of the liver first approach in patients with locally advanced rectal cancer and synchronous metastases. Dis Colon Rectum. 2013;56(3):281-7. doi:10.1097/DCR.0b013e318279b743.
5. Andres A, Toso C, Adam R, et al. A survival analysis of the liver-first reversed management of advanced simultaneous colorectal liver metastases: a LiverMetSurvey-based study. Ann Surg. 2012;256(5):772-8; discussion 778-9. doi: 10.1097/SLA.0b013e3182734423.
6. Yip VS, Collins B, Dunne DFJ, et al. Optimal imaging sequence for staging in colorectal liver metastases: analysis of three hypothetical imaging strategies. Eur J Cancer. 2014; 50:937-43. doi.org/10.1016/j.ejca.2013.11.025.
7. Sahani DV, Bajwa MA, Andrabi Y, et al. Current status of imaging and emerging techniques to evaluate liver metastases from colorectal carcinoma. Ann Surg. 2014;259:861-72. doi:10.1097/SLA.0000000000000525.
8. Lau LF, Williams DS, Lee ST, et al. Metabolic response to preoperative chemotherapy predicts prognosis for patients undergoing surgical resection of colorectal cancer metastatic to the liver. Ann Surg Oncol. 2014;21:2420-8. doi:10.1245/s10434-014-3590-0.

9. Shindoh J, Loyer EM, Kopetz S, et al. Optimal morphologic response to pre-operative chemotherapy: an alternate outcome endpoint before resection of hepatic colorectal metastases. J Clin Oncol. 2012;31:4566-72. doi:10.1200/JCO. 2012.15.2854.

10. Lastoria S, Piccirillo MC, Caraco C, et al. Early PET/CT scan is more effective than RECIST in predicting outcome of patients with liver metastases from colorectal cancer treated with preoperative chemotherapy plus bevacizumab. J Nucl Med. 2013;54(12):2062-9. doi:10.2967/jnumed.113.119909.

11. Wale A, Brown G. A practical review of the performance and interpretation of staging magnetic resonance imaging for rectal cancer. Top Magn Reson Imaging. 2014;23(4): 213-23.

12. Haddad AJ, Bani Hani M, Pawlik TM, et al. Colorectal liver metastases. Int J Surg Oncol. 2011;2011:285840. doi:10.1155/2011/285840.

13. Tanaka K, Murakami T, Yabushita Y, et al. Maximal debulking liver resection as a beneficial treatment strategy for advanced and aggressive colorectal liver metastases. Anticancer Res. 2014;34(10):5547-54.

14. Clark ME, Smith RR. Liver directed therapies in metastatic colorectal cancer. J Gastrointest Oncol. 2014;5(5):374-87. doi:10.3978/j.issn.2078-6891.2014.064.

15. Stumpfle R, Riga A, Deshpande R, et al. Anaesthesia for metastatic liver resection surgery. Current Anaesthesia & Critical Care. 2009;20:3-7. doi: 10.1016/j. cacc.2008.10.009.

16. Nordlinger B, Sorbye H, Glimelius B, et al. EORTC Gastro-Intestinal Tract Cancer Group; Cancer Research UK; Arbeitsgruppe Lebermetastasen und-tumoren in der Chirurgischen Arbeitsgemeinschaft Onkologie (ALM-CAO); Australasian Gastro-Intestinal Trials Group (AGITG); Fédération Francophone de Cancérologie Digestive (FFCD). Perioperative FOLFOX4 chemotherapy and surgery versus surgery alone for resectable liver metastases from colorectal cancer (EORTC 40983): long-term results of a randomised, controlled, phase 3 trial. Lancet Oncol. 2013;14(12):1208-15. doi: 10.1016/S1470-2045(13)70447-9.

17. Folprecht G, Grothey A, Alberts S, et al. Neoadjuvant treatment of unresectable colorectal liver metastases: correlation between tumour response and resection rates.Ann Oncol. 2005;16(8):1311-9. doi:10.1093/annonc/mdi246.

18. Suzuki C, Blomqvist L, Sundin A, et al. The initial change in tumor size predicts response and survival in patients with metastatic colorectal cancer treated with combination chemotherapy.Ann Oncol. 2012;23(4):948-54.

19. Ficorella C, Bruera G, Cannita K, et al. Triplet chemotherapy in patients with metastatic colorectal cancer: towards the best way to safely administer a highly active regimen in clinical practice. Clin Colorectal Cancer. 2012;11(4):229-37. doi:10.1016/j.clcc.2012.05.001.

20. Ychou M, Viret F, Kramar A, et al. Tritherapy with fluorouracil/leucovorin, irinotecan and oxaliplatin (FOLFIRINOX): a phase II study in colorectal cancer patients with non-resectable liver metastases. Cancer Chemother Pharmacol. 2008;62(2):195-201.

21. Saltz LB, Clarke S, Díaz-Rubio E, et al. Bevacizumab in combination with oxali-platin-based chemotherapy as first-line therapy in metastatic colorectal cancer: a randomized phase III study. J Clin Oncol. 2008;26(12):2013-9. doi: 10.1200/JCO.2007.14.9930. [Erratum in: J Clin Oncol. 2008;26(18):3110; J Clin Oncol. 2009 Feb 1;27(4):653.]

22. Hurwitz HI, Tebbutt NC, Kabbinavar F, et al. Efficacy and safety of bevacizumab in metastatic colorectal cancer: pooled analysis from seven randomized controlled trials. Oncologist. 2013;18(9):1004-12. doi: 10.1634/theoncologist.2013-0107.

23. Tanaka K, Ichikawa Y, Endo I. Liver resection for advanced or aggressive colorectal cancer metastases in the era of effective chemotherapy: a review. Int J Clin Oncol. 2011;16:452-63. doi:10.1007/s10147-011-0291-6.

24. Douillard JY, Oliner KS, Siena S, et al. Panitumumab-FOLFOX4 treatment and RAS mutations in colorectal cancer. N Engl J Med. 2013;369(11):1023-34.

25. Bokemeyer C, et al. Treatment outcome according to tumor RAS mutation status in OPUS study patients with metastatic colorectal cancer (mCRC) randomized to FOLFOX4 with/without cetuximab. J Clin Oncol. 2014;32(5s):(suppl; abstr 3505).

26. Ciardiello F, et al. Treatment outcome according to tumor RAS mutation status in CRYSTAL study patients with metastatic colorectal cancer (mCRC) randomized to FOLFIRI with/without cetuximab. J Clin Oncol. 2014;32(5s):(suppl; abstr 3506).

27. Giakoustidis A, Mudan S, Hagemann T. tumour microenvironment: overview with an emphasis on the colorectal liver metastasis pathway. Cancer Microenviron. 2014 Oct 3. doi: 10.1007/s12307-014-0155-5. [Epub ahead of print]

28. Marques AM, Turner A, de Mello RA. Personalising medicine for metastatic colorectal cancer: current developments. World J Gastroenterol. 2014;20(30): 10425-31. doi: 10.3748/wjg.v20.i30.10425.

29. Adam R, De Gramont A, Figueras J, et al; Jean-Nicolas Vauthey of the EGOSLIM (Expert Group on OncoSurgery Management of LIver Metastases) Group. The oncosurgery approach to managing liver metastases from colorectal cancer: a multidisciplinary international consensus. Oncologist. 2012;17(10):1225-39.

30. Stoltz A, Gagnière J, Dupré A, et al. Radiofrequency ablation for colorectal liver metastases. J Visc Surg. 2014;151(Suppl 1):S33-44. doi: 10.1016/j.jviscsurg. 2013.12.005.

31. Correa-Gallego C, Fong Y, Gonen M, et al. A retrospective comparison of microwave ablation vs. radiofrequency ablation for colorectal cancer hepatic metastases. Ann Surg Oncol. 2014 Jun 3. doi: 10.1245/s10434-014-3817-0 [Epub ahead of print]

32. Felekouras E, Petrou A, Neofytou K, et al. Combined ultrasonic aspiration and saline-linked radiofrequency precoagulation. A step toward bloodless liver resection without the need of liver inflow occlusion. Analysis of 313 consecutive patients. World Journal of Surgical oncology. 2014;12:357. doi:10.1186/1477-7819-12-357.

33. Reddy SK, Pawlik TM, Zorzi D, et al. Simultaneous resections of colorectal cancer and synchronous liver metastases: a multi-institutional analysis. Ann Surg Oncol. 2007;14(12):3481-9.

34. Slesser AA, Chand M, Goldin R, et al. Outcomes of simultaneous resections for patients with synchronous colorectal liver metastases. Eur J Surg Oncol. 2013;39(12):1384-93.

35. Slesser AA, Similis C, Goldin R, et al. A meta-analysis comparing simultaneous versus delayed resections in patients with synchronous colorectal liver metastases. Surg Oncol. 2013;22(1):36-47.

36. de Haas RJ, Adam R, Wicherts DA, et al. Comparison of simultaneous or delayed liver surgery for limited synchronous colorectal metastases. Br J Surg. 2010;97(8):1279-89. doi: 10.002/bjs.7106.

37. Seth R, Tai L-H, Falls T, et al. Surgical stress promotes the development of cancer metastases by a coagulation-dependent mechanism involving natural killer cells in a murine model. Ann Surg Oncol. 2013;258:158-68. doi:10.1097/SLA.0b013e31826fcbdb.

38. Gil-Bernabe AM, Lucotti S, Muschel RJ. Coagulation and metastasis: what does the experimental literature tell us? Br J Haematol. 2013;162:433-41. oi:10.1111/bjh.12381.

39. Kaye AD, Patel N, Bueno FR, et al. Effects of opiates, anaesthetic techniques, and other perioperative factors on surgical cancer patients. Ocshner J. 2014;14:216-28.

40. Turrini O, Viret F, Guiramand J, et al. Strategies for the treatment of synchronous liver metastasis. Eur J Surg Oncol. 2007;33(6):735-40.

41. Hillingsø JG, Wille-Jørgensen P. Staged or simultaneous resection of synchronous liver metastases from colorectal cancer—a systematic review. Colorectal Dis. 2009 Jan;11(1):3-10. doi: 10.1111/j.1463-1318.2008.01625.x. [Review. Erratum in: Colorectal Dis. 2009 Jun;11(5):540.]

42. Adam R, Delvart V, Pascal G, et al. Rescue surgery for unresectable colorectal liver metastases downstaged by chemotherapy: a model to predict long-term survival. Ann Surg. 2004;240(4):644-57; discussion 57-8.

43. Wong R, Cunningham D, Barbachano Y, et al. A multicentre study of capecitabine, oxaliplatin plus bevacizumab as perioperative treatment of patients with poor-risk colorectal liver-only metastases not selected for upfront resection. Ann Oncol. 2011;22(9):2042-8. doi: 10.1093/annonc/mdq714.

44. Yoon YS, Kim CW, Lim SB, et al. Palliative surgery in patients with unresectable colorectal liver metastases: a propensity score matching analysis. J Surg Oncol. 2014;109(3):239-44. doi: 10.1002/jso.23480.

45. de Mestier L, Manceau G, Neuzillet C, et al. Primary tumor resection in colorectal cancer with unresectable synchronous metastases: a review. World J Gastrointest Oncol. 2014;6(6):156-69. doi: 10.4251/wjgo.v6.i6.156.

46. Slesser AA, Bhangu A, Brown G, et al. The management of rectal cancer with synchronous liver metastases: a modern surgical dilemma. Tech Coloproctol. 2013;17(1):1-12. doi: 10.1007/s10151-012-0888-4.

47. Alsina J, Choti MA. Liver-directed therapies in colorectal cancer. Semin Oncol. 2011;38(4):561-7.

48. Scorsetti M, Comito T, Tozzi A, et al. Final results of a phase II trial for stereotactic body radiation therapy for patients with inoperable liver metastases from colorectal cancer. J Cancer Res Clin Oncol. 2014 Sep 23. [Epub ahead of print]

49. Hwang M, Jayakrishnan TT, Green DE, et al. Systematic review of outcomes of patients undergoing resection for colorectal liver metastases in the setting of extra hepatic disease. Eur J Cancer. 2014 Jul;50(10):1747-57. doi: 10.1016/j.ejca.2014.03.277.

50. Lam VW, Pang T, Laurence JM, et al. A systematic review of repeat hepatectomy for recurrent colorectal liver metastases. J Gastrointest Surg. 2013;17(7):1312-21. doi: 10.1007/s11605-013-2186-5.

Section
5

Vascular

14

Chapter

Superficial Venous Incompetence and Varicose Vein Management

S Sinha, Toby Richards

INTRODUCTION

Varicose veins are a common pathology affecting between 25% and 40% of the general population.[1,2] Primary varicosities manifesting as engorged, thin-walled veins most commonly arise at the main interconnections between the deep and superficial venous systems: the saphenofemoral junction (SFJ), saphenopopliteal junction (SPJ) and deep perforators. Secondary varicosities are associated with an identifiable pathology (usually in the deep venous system) leading to superficial venous hypertension.[3]

Longitudinal studies suggest that the annual incidence of venous reflux in the general population is almost 1% with the superficial system (in particular the long-saphenous vein) affected in two-thirds of cases.[2] Chronic venous disease secondary to deep venous reflux, obstruction or calf muscle-pump failure can lead to the development of most varicose veins and thus associated risk factors for varicose veins include previous deep venous thrombosis (DVT), posture and raised intra-abdominal pressure (e.g. pregnancy, obesity and intra-abdominal malignancy).[2,3] The Edinburgh Vein Study followed up a random sample of 1,566 men and women aged 18–64 years and found that a past history of DVT and being overweight (body mass index of 25.0–29.9) were associated the development of venous reflux at odds ratios of 11.3 and 2.1, respectively.[2]

Varicose veins can be a significant cause of morbidity with symptomatology independent of objective clinical assessments of severity; having larger varicose veins does not appear to equate to more symptoms and conversely patients with only "minor" apparent varicosities can have significant symptoms.[4] Associated health-care costs in the United Kingdom are significant with treatments for venous disease accounting for approximately 2% of the National Health Service (NHS) budget in 2001.[3] Approximately 90,000 varicose vein operations are performed each year in England.[5]

Objectified assessments of clinical severity of lower limb venous disease allows for delivery of treatment pathways and enables health-care workers to generalise the findings of research units from different countries. The CEAP

(Clinical, Etiology, Anatomy, Pathophysiology) classification is thus commonly used (Table 14.1) although other venous specific (e.g. the Aberdeen Varicose Vein Questionnaire) and generic systems (e.g. Short Form Health Survey 36) are also available to assess quality of life.[3,6,7] A combination of these form the basis of Patient Reported Outcome Measures that the UK Health and Social Care Information Centre use to assess the effectiveness of care delivered to NHS patients undergoing varicose vein surgery.[8]

Table 14.1: CEAP (Clinical, Etiology, Anatomy, Pathophysiology) classification of lower venous disease.

Clinical classification:

C0: No visible or palpable signs of venous disease

C1: Telangiectasies or reticular veins

C2: Varicose veins

C3: Edema

C4a: Pigmentation or eczema

C4b: Lipodermatosclerosis or athrophie blanche

C5: Healed venous ulcer

C6: Active venous ulcer

S: Symptomatic, including ache, pain, tightness, skin irritation, heaviness, and muscle cramps and other complaints attributable to venous dysfunction

A: Asymptomatic

Etiology classification:

Ec: Congenital

Ep: Primary

Es: Secondary

En: No venous cause identified

Anatomic classification:

As: Superficial veins

Ap: Perforating veins

Ad: Deep veins

An: No venous location identified

Pathophysiologic:

Pr: Reflux

Po: Obstruction

Pr,o: Reflux and obstruction

Pn: No venous pathophysiology identifiable

Key Points

- Varicose veins are a common problem particularly in overweight patients.
- Associated health-care costs for managing venous disease are significant.
- Objectified assessments of disease severity and symptomatology allows generalisation of research findings and protocolised treatment.

ROLE OF PREOPERATIVE DUPLEX ULTRASOUND SCANNING (USS)

Historically, preoperative assessment for varicose veins comprised observation with clinical tests such as the "Tourniquet" and "Tap" test occasionally combined with hand-held Doppler examination to determine sites of venous reflux and therefore to direct surgery. These tests are now obsolete—indeed, although the "Tourniquet" and "Tap" tests still feature in medical text books, they should not be used in clinical practice.

Duplex will define the origin of venous reflux causing the varicose veins and will confirm function and patency of the deep venous system. Duplex is superior to both clinical examination and hand-held Doppler for accurate assessment of venous reflux.[9-11] Indeed, although incompetence of the saphenous veins is common, only three-quarters of patients are suitable for endovenous therapy [e.g. due to tortuous or very large calibre (>12 mm) veins, bifid systems, an extra-fascial venous course or pelvic reflux as the origin of venous incompetence].[12] Consequently, surgery for primary varicose veins in the absence of pre-operative Duplex USS imaging may result in inadequate or inappropriate surgery. In a randomized trial, a re-operation rate of 9.5% and recurrent reflux rate of 41.1% for patients was seen in those who did not have pre-operative imaging compared to rates of 1.4% and 15.0% in those who did.[13] Thus guidance in both the UK and USA now recommends Duplex USS imaging as standard for preoperative assessment in all patients with varicose veins.[14,15]

SURGICAL AND CLOSURE TECHNIQUES

Open Surgery

First described by Friedrich von Trendelenburg more than 200 years ago, open surgery was the "gold standard" technique for operative management of lower limb varicose veins. The underlying principle remains to disconnect the point of reflux from the deep venous system into the superficial system. Indeed, the Trendelenburg operation of ligation of the long saphenous vein (LSV) at the femoral vein continued as "normal" practise into the

1980s. This evolved to flush ligation of the LSV at the SFJ in an attempt to reduce neovascularisation and recurrent reflux. Attempts to seal the SFJ or cover this with a synthetic patch and prevent recurrence by neovascularisation proved ineffectual and were abandoned.[16] Addition of LSV stripping to the knee developed into routine practice with observational evidence of reduced need for re-intervention.[17] SFJ flush ligation and stripping of the LSV remains the standard of surgical care in many centres.

However, the last decade has seen the development of minimally invasive endovenous techniques and has led to a 50% reduction in the proportion of venous interventions performed as open surgery in England.[3] The National Institute for Health and Clinical Excellence in the United Kingdom has recently recommended endothermal ablation as the first-line treatment of choice in patients with varicose veins.[15]

Endovenous Techniques

Endovenous approaches rely on injuring the target vein endothelium and application of compression to stimulate occlusion of the lumen. The most common techniques in current clinical usage are endothermal ablation (by either laser or radiofrequency, RF) and chemical ablation with foam sclerosant. All of these techniques require accurate pre-procedural duplex scanning to define the exact venous segment to be treated and are performed under ultrasound control to determine accuracy and effect of the intervention. In many cases procedures can be performed under local anaesthetic and in the outpatient setting.

Endothermal Ablation

The technique for either laser or radiofrequency ablation (RFA) is similar.

Ultrasound guidance is used to facilitate vein cannulation using a Seldinger technique and a standard (often 7fr) introducer sheath. Placement of the catheter is confirmed with USS along the target vein to the origin of reflux (usually 2 cm distal to the SFJ or SPJ). USS is then used to guide instillation of saline with local anaesthetic agent (commonly 20 mL 1% lidocaine in 500 mL normal saline) around and along the length of the vein within its fascial sheath. This "tumescence" achieves not only anaesthesia but provides a "heat sink" effect to prevent excess heat energy being imparted to surrounding tissues, increases the distance between the vein and the overlying skin (thus reducing the chance of skin burns) and provides latent compression (thus reducing the amount of energy needed to achieve closure). A minimum 1 cm of tumescence around the vein reduces risk of skin burn or fibrosis (which can cause causing postoperative tattoing and "tethering" of the skin). With the patient in "head down" position to empty the vein, the thermal catheter then heat treats the section of vein. Post-procedure the patient is placed into compression for 5–21 days. Complications of the procedure include bruising and superficial thrombophlebitis often several days following intervention. This is usually self-limiting and is managed with conservative therapy of compression and a course of nonsteroidal anti-inflammatory drugs. In the mid-term, some patients have a sense of pulling or tethering in the thigh where the residual LSV fibroses but skin staining, thermal burns or deep venous injury/thrombosis are rare.[3]

Endovenous Laser Ablation (EVLA)

EVLA utilises an optical fibre, normally in the infrared portion of the spectrum, to generate thermal energy (up to 800°C) causing obliteration of the vein and subsequent fibrosis (http://venacure-evlt.com/endovenous-laser-vein-treatment/angiodynamics/products/laser/).[18,19] The term endovenous laser therapy is often confused with EVLA: it is the same treatment but refers to a specific make of 910 nm generator and laser fibre made by Diomed. There are now a variety of fibres with different wavelengths available (from 810 nm to 1470 nm) depending on the manufacturer. Following vein cannulation and subsequent tumescence the laser fibre is withdrawn in a steady continuous manner (0.2 cm/s) whilst discharging a 14W power source with an aim to deliver 60–70 J of energy to each treated centimetre of vein. Complications of the procedure include bruising, skin staining, thermal burns, superficial thrombophlebitis and deep venous injury/thrombosis.[3]

Radiofrequency Ablation

RFA utilises RF waves to generate thermal energy (of 85°C–120°C) instead of laser.[20] Procedural steps for this approach are otherwise as for EVLA. The commonest RFA catheter used is the VNUS ClosureFast system (now known as Venefit, Covidien, Mansfield, MA, USA) (https://www.venefit-procedure.com/closurefast.aspx).[21] VNUS ClosureFast allows deliver of RF energy to a pre-defined length of vein segment (3–7 cm depending on the type of RFA catheter) over 20 seconds with each more distal vein segment treated in subsequent serial 20 second bursts. VNUS ClosureFast facilitates a faster treatment rate (0.35 cm/s) and by allowing discrete segmental treatment, possibly avoids variations in the amount of delivered energy related to operator technique.[3] Other manufacturers of RFA catheters utilise a continuous pull-back technique similar to EVLA.

Sclerotherapy

This technique utilises chemicals, which are toxic to endothelium, to induce venous scarring and subsequent occlusion. In the United Kingdom, 1–3% sodium tetradecyl sulphate (STD) or 0.5–3% polidocanol (PD) are most commonly used. Sclerotherapy is the gold standard for treatment of thread or spider veins by direct injection with microfine needles (31g). It is also used in the treatment of arteriovenous and lymphatic malformations.

For the treatment of varicose veins, STD or PD are emulsified with air in a 1:4 ratio by the Tessari technique using 2 Luer-lock syringes connected by a three-way tap[22] (https://www.youtube.com/watch?v=Zoond6y2dQ0).[23] This converts the sclerosant from a liquid state to a foam. Foam sclerotherapy (FS) is beneficial for three reasons: firstly, it generates a bright ultrasonic signal and can therefore be tracked throughout the treated venous segment (thus also reducing the likelihood of embolisation into the deep venous system), secondly, it achieves greater surface contact with the vein wall and thirdly, it is less prone to deactivation through contact with blood proteins thus increasing its potency. FS can be used to treat either truncal disease or isolated varicosities and has the advantage of being able to navigate tortuous pathways and treat small veins. It is injected into the target vein under US guidance (without the need for tumescent anaesthesia) and, as with EVLA, post-procedural compression is required. Complications of FS include brown skin staining and rarely necrosis (particularly if sclerosant extravasates) as well as DVT and migraine.[3] Neurological events such as transient ischemic attack are rare and it is postulated that they are related to sclerosant or air emboli reaching the cerebral carotid circulation in patients with undiagnosed right-to-left cardiac shunts (e.g. patent foramen ovale).[24,25]

Other Endovenous Ablative Methods

Newer approaches with a smaller (but growing) evidence base than the three aforementioned techniques include steam ablation [Steam Varicose System, which provides thermal ablation through pulsated steam (http://www.inycom.com/productos-medicina/ablacion-endovenosa-por-vapor-de-agua)], non-thermal techniques, which obviate the need for tumescent anaesthesia such as mechanochemical ablation [ClariVein, which uses a rotating wire at the catheter tip to abrade the endothelium and simultaneously delivers intra-luminal sclerosant (http://clarivein.com/)] and intra-luminal adhesive sealant [Sapheon Venaseal Closure System (http://www.venaseal.com/how-venaseal-works/)] as well as hybrid open/endoluminal approaches such as cryoablation.[3,26-32]

Key Points

- Endovenous closure techniques are now established as the preferred treatment for varicose veins.
- Endovenous techniques can be divided into thermal (requiring local anaesthesia) and non-thermal ablative methods.

EFFICACY AND COST-EFFECTIVENESS OF ENDOVENOUS TECHNIQUES

Given the traditional role of open surgery, newer endovenous approaches [especially EVLA, RFA and USS-guided FS (UGFS)] have been subject to scrutiny through numerous randomized controlled trials (RCTs) and subsequent meta-analyses to demonstrate their efficacy.

A recent systematic review identified 28 RCTs suitable for meta-analysis.[33] Eleven RCTs compared EVLA with surgery, 8 RCTs compared RFA with surgery, 4 RCTs compared UGFS with surgery, 5 RCTs compared RFA with EVLA and there was one multi-comparison RCT. Only 3 RCTs were considered to be at low risk of bias.[34-36] The primary outcome was defined as "primary failure" (i.e. failure to completely abolish truncal reflux). As illustrated in Figures 14.1A to D, no difference was found between either RFA or EVLA versus surgery or between RFA and EVLA. UGFS was associated with a greater than two-fold risk of failure in comparison with open surgery. For secondary outcomes, no difference was noted between either RFA or EVLA versus surgery in terms of clinical recurrence whilst EVLA and RFA were associated with significantly less post-operative pain and a lower risk of wound infection and haematoma. RFA conferred a higher risk of post-operative superficial thrombophlebitis in comparison to open surgery (RR 2.3) but was nonetheless associated with a faster return to normal activities (whilst EVLA was not for either outcome). Of note, a homogenous finding within both this meta-analysis and more recent double-blinded RCTs was that postoperative pain after RFA was less in comparison to EVLA.[33,37]

The REACTIV (**R**andomised clinical trial, obs**E**rvational study and **A**ssessment of **C**ost-effec**TI**veness of the treatment of **V**aricose veins) trial had previously demonstrated both the clinical effectiveness and the cost-effectiveness of open surgical intervention in comparison to conservative management.[38] In this context, the cost-effectiveness of newer endovenous techniques in comparison to open surgery has been the subject of considerable interest especially given the current economic climate affecting the NHS.[39] Cost-effectiveness studies suggest that open surgery performed as a day-case and RFA or EVLA performed under local anaesthetic in a day-case or office-based setting are likely to be cost-effective treatments whilst the overall utility of UGFS remains uncertain as its initial lower cost may be offset by the higher costs of re-intervention in the medium term.[40,41]

VENOUS ULCERATION

Approximately 3% of patients with varicose veins will develop venous ulcers.[15] However, what is not clear is who will get ulceration—indeed many patients can have varicose veins for years without any impact on their quality of life.

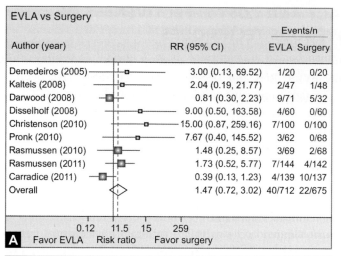

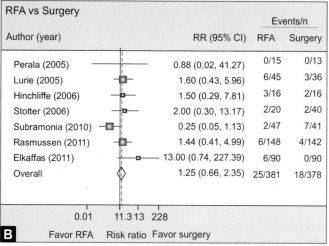

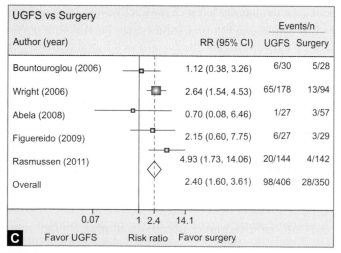

Figs. 14.1A to C

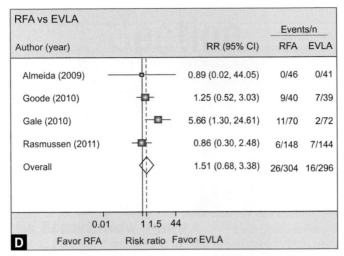

Figs. 14.1A to D: Meta-analysis of pooled results for primary outcome (failure to completely abolish truncal reflux) after different interventions.
Source: Reproduced with permission from Siribumrungwong B, Noorit P, Wilasrusmee C, Attia J, Thakkinstian A. A systematic review and meta-analysis of randomised controlled trials comparing endovenous ablation and surgical intervention in patients with varicose vein. Eur J Vasc Endovasc Surg. 2012;44(2):214-23.

The impact of venous ulceration is significant: the average healing time is 8 weeks with a 60–80% relapse rate and 10–20% of patients are poor responders requiring prolonged (often more than 12 months) labour-intensive nursing care (Fig. 14.2).[42] The financial burden of venous ulcer care is estimated at $3 billion annually across Western countries. In the United Kingdom, wound management (of all descriptions) represents the majority of clinical activity performed by district (community) nurses. The accepted treatment for venous ulceration is compression either delivered via layered bandaging or from elasticated stockings.[3,43] The ESCHAR study (**E**ffect of **S**urgery and **C**ompression on **H**ealing **A**nd **R**ecurrence) randomised 500 patients with active or recently healed venous ulceration to either compression alone or compression with superficial venous surgery.[44] Although rates of wound healing were no different (hazard ratio 0.84; 95% confidence interval, CI, 0.77 to 1.24), ulcer recurrence rates were significantly reduced in the group undergoing surgery (hazard ratio -2.76; 95% CI -1.78 to -4.27)—an effect, which persisted at four years.[44,45] Trials are currently ongoing to compare early versus delayed intervention in lower limb venous ulceration [e.g. the EVRA (**E**arly **V**enous **R**eflux **A**blation) Ulcer trial; http://public.ukcrn.org.uk/Search/StudyDetail.aspx?StudyID=15078].[46]

COMPRESSION HOSIERY

Compression was considered a first-line treatment for symptomatic but otherwise uncomplicated varicose veins as they are non-invasive and

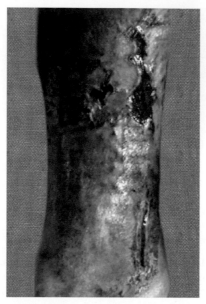

Fig. 14.2: Venous ulceration affecting the gaiter area.
Source: Reproduced with permission from Onida S, Lane TRA, Davies AH. Varicose veins and their management. Surgery—Oxford International Edition. 2013;31(5):211-7.

cost-effective.[3] The mechanism of action of compression is through the exertion of graded external pressure to the skin at the level of the ankle and at sequentially lower amounts as one ascends higher. The net result is a reduction in the volume of the venous reservoir, reduced venous stasis/reflux, improved capillary pressure gradients and thus improved arterial inflow.[3] There are five different classification types for compression hosiery and each type has between three and four classes of compression representing different in vitro pressure measurements.[47] In the United Kingdom, class II stockings (British Standard), which exert a pressure of 18–24 mm Hg are most commonly prescribed.[3]

Due to study heterogeneity (e.g. the use of different types of stockings in different patient groups across different studies) and consequently poor-quality evidence, the scientific basis supporting the use of compression hosiery for uncomplicated varicose veins is equivocal and current official guidance in both the USA and the United Kingdom suggests that compression should not be used as a rationing tool in lieu of definitive treatment.[3,14,15,47]

RECURRENCE AND PELVIC VEIN REFLUX

Recurrence after varicose vein surgery is relatively common, associated with poorer patient outcomes and can present with advanced clinical signs (skin changes) in a quarter of patients.[48] Treatment is frequently challenging

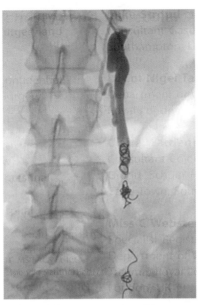

Fig. 14.3: Embolization of the left ovarian vein with contrast demonstrating reflux from the left renal vein.

because of the atypical anatomy of recurrence and the hazards associated with re-operative fields.[49] Knowledge of the history and operations undertaken for varicose veins is therefore necessary to optimise outcomes and consequently the surgeon should be aware of the index procedures to help guide future definitive treatment.

The term "REVAS" (**RE**current **V**arices **A**fter **S**urgery) was proposed by international consensus to define: true recurrences (e.g. due to neovascularisation), residual veins [either due to tactical error (inappropriate initial surgery) or technical error (inadequate surgical technique)] and new varices as a result of disease progression.[48,50] In 10% of cases, no source of reflux can be demonstrated but in the remainder the majority (50%) of recurrence is due to SFJ incompetence whilst a further 20% have pelvic or abdominal vein reflux.[48,51] Intervention to abdominal and pelvic veins is emerging as a neoadjunctive treatment (i.e. prior to lower limb venous surgery) in the management of patients with lower limb varicose veins demonstrated to have pelvic vein reflux on preoperative imaging (Fig. 14.3).[52]

In women with a pelvic component to their lower limb venous insufficiency, focussed questioning and examination at consultation will usually suggest a pelvic source. Thus the presence of varicosities of the vulva (particularly in pregnancy), atypical leg symptoms (typically mid-thigh pain) and also lower limb venous symptoms that vary with the menstrual cycle are suggestive whilst atypical medial or posterior position of the varicose veins may also be observed.[53,54]

Treatment by embolisation of incompetent pelvic veins has been shown to reduce the risk of lower limb varicose vein recurrence. Indeed, Creton et al. observed an improvement in 80% of cases of recurrent varicose veins three years postembolisation of incompetent ovarian and pelvic varices.[55] Similar results have been reported by van der Vleuten et al. who noted an improvement of symptoms in 66.9% of patients two months after embolisation.[56] Meneses et al. investigated the effects of performing embolisation before recurrent varicose vein surgery in a small series and found that embolisation both reduced the risk of re-recurrence and improved symptoms even without surgery.[57]

Key Points

- Numerous randomized studies have confirmed the efficacy of endovenous techniques in comparison to open surgery.
- Venous ulceration is the most severe complication of varicose disease and confers a significant disease burden due to prolonged healing times and high relapse rates.
- Compression has been demonstrated to accelerate healing of venous ulceration whilst surgery has not.
- Adjunctive techniques such as abolition of pelvic vein reflux may have a role in reducing recurrence of varicose veins.

CONCLUSION

The modern management of patients with varicose veins focuses on the patients' symptoms and clinical severity of disease. Accurate diagnosis by routine preoperative duplex ultrasound will enable direction of appropriate therapy and should be considered mandatory. In most cases, treatment can be delivered through new endovenous modalities thus obviating the need for hospital admission. Most patients can ambulate within hours, analgesic requirements are minimal and many return to work within days. Accurate diagnosis of the origin of the varicosities and a treatment plan, which addresses these sources, will minimise the risk of recurrence.

REFERENCES

1. Beebe-Dimmer JL, Pfeifer JR, Engle JS, et al. The epidemiology of chronic venous insufficiency and varicose veins. Ann Epidemiol. 2005;15(3):175-84.
2. Robertson LA, Evans CJ, Lee AJ, et al. Incidence and risk factors for venous reflux in the general population: Edinburgh Vein Study. Eur J Vasc Endovasc Surg. 2014;48(2):208-14.
3. Onida S, Lane TRA, Davies AH. Varicose veins and their management. Surgery—Oxford International Edition. 2013;31(5):211-7.

4. Darvall KA, Bate GR, Adam DJ, et al. Generic health-related quality of life is significantly worse in varicose vein patients with lower limb symptoms independent of CEAP clinical grade. Eur J Vasc Endovasc Surg. 2012;44(3):341-4.

5. Gohel MS, Davies AH. Varicose veins: highlighting the confusion over how and where to treat. Eur J Vasc Endovasc Surg. 2008;36(1):107-8.

6. Porter JM, Moneta GL. Reporting standards in venous disease: an update. International Consensus Committee on Chronic Venous Disease. J Vasc Surg. 1995;21(4):635-45.

7. Eklof B, Rutherford RB, Bergan JJ, et al. Revision of the CEAP classification for chronic venous disorders: consensus statement. J Vasc Surg. 2004;40(6): 1248-52.

8. Health and Social Care Information Centre. Background information about PROMs. [online] Available from: http://www.hscic.gov.uk/article/3843/Background-information-about-PROMs. [Accessed Sep 23, 2014].

9. Singh S, Lees TA, Donlon M, et al. Improving the preoperative assessment of varicose veins. Br J Surg. 1997;84(6):801-2.

10. Wills V, Moylan D, Chambers J. The use of routine duplex scanning in the assessment of varicose veins. Aust N Z J Surg. 1998;68(1):41-4.

11. Mercer KG, Scott DJ, Berridge DC. Preoperative duplex imaging is required before all operations for primary varicose veins. Br J Surg. 1998;85(11):1495-7.

12. Goode SD, Kuhan G, Altaf N, et al. Suitability of varicose veins for endovenous treatments. Cardiovasc Intervent Radiol. 2009; 32(5):988-91.

13. Blomgren L, Johansson G, Bergqvist D. Randomized clinical trial of routine preoperative duplex imaging before varicose vein surgery. Br J Surg. 2005;92(6): 688-94.

14. Gloviczki P, Comerota AJ, Dalsing MC, et al. The care of patients with varicose veins and associated chronic venous diseases: clinical practice guidelines of the Society for Vascular Surgery and the American Venous Forum. J Vasc Surg. 2011;53(5 Suppl):2S-48S.

15. Marsden G, Perry M, Kelley K, et al. Diagnosis and management of varicose veins in the legs: summary of NICE guidance. BMJ. 2013;347:f4279.

16. Bhatti TS, Whitman B, Harradine K, et al. Causes of re-recurrence after polytetrafluoroethylene patch saphenoplasty for recurrent varicose veins. Br J Surg. 2000;87(10):1356-60.

17. Dwerryhouse S, Davies B, Harradine K, et al. Stripping the long saphenous vein reduces the rate of reoperation for recurrent varicose veins: five-year results of a randomized trial. J Vasc Surg. 1999;29(4):589-92.

18. Navarro L, Min RJ, Bone C. Endovenous laser: a new minimally invasive method of treatment for varicose veins--preliminary observations using an 810 nm diode laser. Dermatol Surg. 2001;27(2):117-22.

19. http://venacure-evlt.com/endovenous-laser-vein-treatment/angiodynamics/products/laser/. [Accessed Sep 23, 2014].

20. Goldman MP. Closure of the greater saphenous vein with endoluminal radiofrequency thermal heating of the vein wall in combination with ambulatory phlebectomy: preliminary 6-month follow-up. Dermatol Surg. 2000;26(5):452-6.

21. https://www.venefitprocedure.com/closurefast.aspx. [Accessed Sep 23, 2014].

22. Tessari L, Cavezzi A, Frullini A. Preliminary experience with a new sclerosing foam in the treatment of varicose veins. Dermatol Surg. 2001;27(1):58-60.

23. https://www.youtube.com/watch?v=Zoond6y2dQ0. [Accessed Sep 23, 2014].

24. Sarvananthan T, Shepherd AC, Willenberg T, et al. Neurological complications of sclerotherapy for varicose veins. J Vasc Surg. 2012;55(1):243-51.

25. Forlee MV, Grouden M, Moore DJ, et al. Stroke after varicose vein foam injection sclerotherapy. J Vasc Surg. 2006;43(1):162-4.

26. Mueller RL, Raines JK. Clari Vein mechanochemical ablation: background and procedural details. Vasc Endovascular Surg. 2013;47(3):195-206.

27. Lawson J, Gauw S, van Vlijmen C, et al. Sapheon: the solution? Phlebology. 2013;28(Suppl 1):2-9.

28. van den Bos RR, Malskat WS, De Maeseneer MG, et al. Randomized clinical trial of endovenous laser ablation versus steam ablation (LAST trial) for great saphenous varicose veins. Br J Surg. 2014;101(9):1077-83.

29. van den Bos RR, Milleret R, Neumann M, et al. Proof-of-principle study of steam ablation as novel thermal therapy for saphenous varicose veins. J Vasc Surg. 2011;53(1):181-6.

30. http://www.inycom.com/productos-medicina/ablacion-endovenosa-por-vapor-de-agua. [Accessed Sep 23, 2014].

31. http://clarivein.com/. [Accessed Sep 23, 2014].

32. http://www.venaseal.com/how-venaseal-works/. [Accessed Sep 23, 2014].

33. Siribumrungwong B, Noorit P, Wilasrusmee C, et al. A systematic review and meta-analysis of randomised controlled trials comparing endovenous ablation and surgical intervention in patients with varicose vein. Eur J Vasc Endovasc Surg. 2012;44(2):214-23.

34. Subramonia S, Lees T. Randomized clinical trial of radiofrequency ablation or conventional high ligation and stripping for great saphenous varicose veins. Br J Surg. 2010;97(3):328-36.

35. de Medeiros CA, Luccas GC. Comparison of endovenous treatment with an 810 nm laser versus conventional stripping of the great saphenous vein in patients with primary varicose veins. Dermatol Surg. 2005;31(12):1685-94; discussion 94.

36. Almeida JI, Kaufman J, Gockeritz O, et al. Radiofrequency endovenous ClosureFAST versus laser ablation for the treatment of great saphenous reflux: a multicenter, single-blinded, randomized study (RECOVERY study). J Vasc Interv Radiol. 2009;20(6):752-9.

37. Nordon IM, Hinchliffe RJ, Brar R, et al. A prospective double-blind randomized controlled trial of radiofrequency versus laser treatment of the great saphenous vein in patients with varicose veins. Ann Surg. 2011;254(6):876-81.

38. Michaels JA, Campbell WB, Brazier JE, et al. Randomised clinical trial, obser-vational study and assessment of cost-effectiveness of the treatment of varicose veins (REACTIV trial). Health Technol Assess. 2006;10(13):1-196, iii-iv.

39. Gohel M. Which treatments are cost-effective in the management of varicose veins? Phlebology. 2013;28(Suppl 1):153-7.

40. Carroll C, Hummel S, Leaviss J, et al. Clinical effectiveness and cost-effectiveness of minimally invasive techniques to manage varicose veins: a systematic review and economic evaluation. Health Technol Assess. 2013;17(48):i-xvi, 1-141.

41. Gohel MS, Epstein DM, Davies AH. Cost-effectiveness of traditional and end-ovenous treatments for varicose veins. Br J Surg. 2010;97(12):1815-23.

42. Eberhardt RT, Raffetto JD. Chronic venous insufficiency. Circulation. 201422; 130(4):333-46.

43. Stucker M, Link K, Reich-Schupke S, et al. Compression and venous ulcers. Phlebology. 2013;28(Suppl 1):68-72.

44. Barwell JR, Davies CE, Deacon J, et al. Comparison of surgery and compression with compression alone in chronic venous ulceration (ESCHAR study): randomised controlled trial. Lancet. 2004;363(9424):1854-9.

45. Gohel MS, Barwell JR, Taylor M, et al. Long term results of compression therapy alone versus compression plus surgery in chronic venous ulceration (ESCHAR): randomised controlled trial. BMJ. 2007; 335(7610):83.

46. http://public.ukcrn.org.uk/Search/StudyDetail.aspx?StudyID=15078. [Accessed Sep 23, 2014].

47. Palfreyman SJ, Michaels JA. A systematic review of compression hosiery for uncomplicated varicose veins. Phlebology. 2009;24(Suppl 1):13-33.

48. Brake M, Lim CS, Shepherd AC, et al. Pathogenesis and etiology of recurrent varicose veins. J Vasc Surg. 2013;57(3):860-8.

49. De Maeseneer M. Surgery for recurrent varicose veins: toward a less-invasive approach? Perspect Vasc Surg Endovasc Ther. 2011;23(4):244-9.

50. Perrin MR, Labropoulos N, Leon LR, Jr. Presentation of the patient with recurrent varices after surgery (REVAS). J Vasc Surg. 2006;43(2):327-34; discussion 34.

51. Marsh P, Holdstock J, Harrison C, et al. Pelvic vein reflux in female patients with varicose veins: comparison of incidence between a specialist private vein clinic and the vascular department of a National Health Service District General Hospital. Phlebology. 2009;24(3):108-13.

52. Ratnam LA, Marsh P, Holdstock JM, et al. Pelvic vein embolisation in the management of varicose veins. Cardiovasc Intervent Radiol. 2008;31(6):1159-64.

53. Asciutto G, Asciutto KC, Mumme A, et al. Pelvic venous incompetence: reflux patterns and treatment results. Eur J Vasc Endovasc Surg. 2009;38(3):381-6.

54. Asciutto G, Mumme A, Asciutto KC, et al. Pelvic vein incompetence influences pain levels in patients with lower limb varicosity. Phlebology. 2010;25(4):179-83.

55. Creton D, Hennequin L, Kohler F, et al. Embolisation of symptomatic pelvic veins in women presenting with non-saphenous varicose veins of pelvic origin—three-year follow-up. Eur J Vasc Endovasc Surg. 2007;34(1):112-7.

56. van der Vleuten CJ, van Kempen JA, Schultze-Kool LJ. Embolization to treat pelvic congestion syndrome and vulval varicose veins. Int J Gynaecol Obstet. 2012;118(3):227-30.

57. Meneses L, Fava M, Diaz P, et al. Embolization of incompetent pelvic veins for the treatment of recurrent varicose veins in lower limbs and pelvic congestion syndrome. Cardiovasc Intervent Radiol. 2013; 36(1):128-32.

Section
6

Clinical
Trials

A Review of Recent Randomised Controlled Trials in Surgery

Siân Pugh, Nicholas Jenkins

OESOPHAGOGASTRIC

Bariatric Surgery

Treatment options for obesity include non-surgical treatments, such as behavioural therapies, dietary changes and pharmacotherapies and bariatric surgery. Current National Institute for Clinical Excellence guidelines recommend evaluation of bariatric surgery for individuals with a body mass index (BMI) >40 or >35 with serious comorbidities related to obesity in whom all appropriate non-surgical measures have been tried.[1]

The most common surgical techniques used are Roux-en-Y gastric bypass, sleeve gastrectomy or gastric banding. Two RCTs were reported in 2013 comparing operative to nonoperative treatment strategies. The Diabetes Surgery Study compared the efficacy of intensive medical management (included weight lowering medications) to Roux-en-Y gastric bypass surgery to achieve control of comorbid risk factors in patients with diabetes.[2] After 12 months, 28 participants (49%; 95% confidence interval, CI, 36%–63%) in the gastric bypass group and 11 (19% 95%CI 10%–32%) in the lifestyle-medical management group had achieved the primary endpoints of HbA1c <7.0%, LDL cholesterol < 100 mg/dL and systolic blood pressure <130 mm Hg (odds ratios, OR, 4·8; 95%CI 1·9–11·7). The other study randomised obese participants (BMI >28) with type II diabetes and hypertension into three groups of usual care, usual care with exenatide, a glucagon-like peptide-1 agonist and Roux-en-Y gastric bypass surgery.[3] The study found that participants in the group randomised to surgery had the greatest improvement in the primary endpoint, left ventricular mass index as a measure of cardiac function, at 12 months. BMI was also maximally reduced in the group undergoing surgery.

A meta-analysis of 11 studies, including the above two RCTs, aimed to quantify the overall effects of bariatric surgery compared to non-surgical treatment for obesity.[4] The authors found that surgery resulted in a greater weight loss (mean difference -26 kg (95%CI -31 to -21)) and higher remission rates of type II diabetes [relative risk 22·1 (3·2 to 154·3)]. As with the two RCTs above, follow-up in all trials was short and overall limited to a maximum of two years. As such information on the longer term efficacy of these interventions is lacking.

Key Point

- Bariatric surgery is an effective treatment for obesity although the long-term efficacy is yet to be evaluated.

Gastro-oesophageal Reflux Disease

The REFLUX trial compared minimal access surgery to medical management for gastro-oesophageal reflux disease with longer follow-up data available to determine whether benefits are sustained.[5] The primary outcome measure was self-reported quality-of-life score on disease-specific REFLUX questionnaire. Just 63% (112/178) of those allocated to surgery actually underwent an operation, which likely reflects the difficulty in randomising between two very different treatments. Despite this there were still clear differences in outcome between the intention to treat groups with the RELFUX score significantly favouring the surgical treatment group (mean difference 8·5 95%CI 3·9–13·1 $p < ·001$, at five years).

Key Point

- The improved outcome from surgical treatment of gastro-oesophageal reflux disease compared to medical management was sustained at five years follow-up.

HEPATOPANCREATOBILIARY

Enhanced Recovery Following Liver Resection

Enhanced recovery pathways (ERPs) after surgery aim to attenuate the stress response to surgery and enable a rapid recovery. To date there is limited evidence for their use following liver resection. A small RCT was conducted in one UK hospital comparing an ERP after open liver resection to standard care.[6] The trial was powered to detect an ambitious three-day reduction in length of stay with 46 patients in the ERP group and 45 in the standard care group included in the analysis. Median time until medically fit for discharge was reduced in the ERP group (three vs six days with standard care; $p < ·001$), as was length of stay (four vs seven days; $p < ·001$).

Although these results reach significance the study does have limitations. Instead of using distance randomisation, the sealed envelope system was used, which can compromise this process.[7] There was no stratification resulting in an imbalance in baseline characteristics between the groups with more patients in the ERP group having higher Portsmouth modification of the P-POSSUM operative severity scores, reflecting the higher number of major resections in this group ($p = \cdot012$). The median length of stay achieved in both groups of this study are certainly excellent and may reflect health-care professionals being more attuned to the principles of enhanced recovery and therefore incorporating aspects into all patients' management.

Key Point

- Enhanced recovery pathways, which are increasingly being adopted for general surgical procedures, are both safe and effective to use after liver resection.

Ischaemia Reperfusion Injury

The main disadvantage of vascular inflow occlusion used during liver surgery to reduce bleeding is the postoperative liver dysfunction and morbidity that can result from ischaemia-reperfusion injury. Two meta-analyses published in 2013 focused on therapeutic strategies to reduce the effects of such ischaemia-reperfusion injury. The first examined RCTs evaluating ischaemic preconditioning prior to either continuous or intermittent clamping.[8] Eleven suitable studies were identified, but no significant benefit was found in terms of mortality or morbidity; however, the trials identified were somewhat heterogeneous.

A further meta-analysis aimed to determine the effect of administration of perioperative steroids on ischaemia-reperfusion injury and the surgical stress response.[9] Six studies were included, of which five were RCT's, and the pooled results demonstrated that patients receiving intravenous glucocorticoids were 24 per cent less likely to suffer postoperative morbidity compared with controls (risk ratio $0\cdot76$, 95%CI $0\cdot57–0\cdot99$; $p = \cdot047$). It is unlikely that this will be incorporated into clinical practice since the study has a number of limitations including that less than one fifth of study subjects underwent major hepatectomy.

Pancreaticoduodenectomy

Pancreaticoduodenectomy (PD) is the only therapeutic modality offering long-term survival in patients with operable pancreatic head or periampullary tumours. It remains a surgical procedure with high morbidity often related to the pancreatic anastomosis. The postoperative course can be substantially affected by the occurrence of pancreatic fistula potentially leading to the life-threatening complication of a delayed bleed from a pseudoaneurysm. Much research has addressed the optimum approach to pancreatic anastomosis although there is still little consensus.

Two trials were published in 2013 favouring reconstruction with pancreaticogastrostomy (PG) over pancreaticojejunostomy (PJ).[10,11] One randomised 329 patients intraoperatively to either PG or PJ after PD for pancreatic or periampullary tumours.[10] Patients were stratified according to size of pancreatic duct measured intraoperatively. Whilst the overall incidence of postoperative complications did not differ between the groups, there was a significant difference in the primary outcome measure of clinical postoperative pancreatic fistula (grade B or C as defined by the International Study Group on Pancreatic Fistula). A total of 33 (19·8%) patients in the PJ group and 13 (8·0%) in the PG group had clinical postoperative pancreatic fistula (OR 2·86, 95%CI 1·38–6·17; p = ·002).

A smaller RCT of 123 patients conducted across two centres similarly randomised between PJ and PG intraoperatively without stratification by duct size.[11] The primary endpoint of the study was the incidence and severity of pancreatic fistula after PD. This trial, with slightly different methodologies and inclusion criteria to the first, similarly demonstrated a higher incidence of pancreatic fistula following PJ than for PG (20/58 vs 10/65, respectively; p = ·014). The severity of pancreatic fistula was also higher in the PJ group (grade A: 2% vs 5%; grade B–C: 33% vs 11%; p = ·006).

Whilst the results of both of these RCTs favour PG, the study designs have been questioned.[12,13] Specifically, issues regarding surgeon's experience and the effect of institution volume on outcomes have been raised. In the first trial, surgeons were required to have previously undertaken just five PJ and five PG procedures, whereas the second did not make a stipulation. Neither reported on the annual volume of the participating surgeons nor institutions. Such studies will always be open to criticism and it is noteworthy that whilst the first study is criticised for not standardising the technique of anastomosis, the second is criticised for only allowing a duct-to-mucosa technique in the PJ arm.

Key Point

- There have now been a number of RCTs addressing the optimum pancreatic anastomosis after PD. Current evidence supports the use of PG, however, until there is multi-institutional consensus on the optimum study design it is unlikely that the results of trials will be translated into clinical practice.

Cholecystectomy

Studies on single incision laparoscopic cholecystectomy appear regularly in the literature, although, owing to limited data on the safety of the procedure, it has not been routinely adopted. One particular meta-analysis published in 2013 included 13 RCTs comparing single incision laparoscopic surgery

(SILS) cholecystectomy to the standard laparoscopic approach.[14] There was a higher procedure failure rate, longer operating time, and greater blood loss in the SILS group than the conventional laparoscopic cholecystectomy group. This may in part reflect the fact that in the majority of RCTs included, the SILS procedures were performed during the surgeon's learning curve. Whilst there was no difference found in postoperative pain, cosmetic satisfaction was greater in the SILS group; the authors note these results must be interpreted with caution due to wide confidence intervals and small numbers of RCTs examining some of these outcomes.

Another study evaluated the benefit of the open technique compared to the laparoscopic approach. Patients were randomised to either small incision open cholecystectomy (SIOC), with a 4–8-cm-long transverse incision over the right rectus abdominis muscle, or conventional laparoscopic cholecystectomy.[15] This was a pragmatic expertise-based study with the aim of avoiding the confounder identified in the above meta-analysis that of the surgeon's learning curve. As such, patients were randomised to surgeons with expertise in either intervention, rather than to procedures done by surgeons expected to have equal competence in both operations. Whilst mean duration of surgery was shorter in the SIOC group, there was a small decrease in postoperative quality of life in the SIOC group. Details of what this related to, e.g. cosmesis, are not provided.

Key Point

- Single-incision laparoscopic cholecystectomy is associated with improved cosmetic satisfaction, but there are still no adequately powered trials to assess its safety.

COLORECTAL

Colonic Investigations

Several procedures are available to investigate patients with symptoms suggestive of colorectal cancer. The first randomised data on symptomatic patients were published in 2013 from two trials led by the UK Special Interest Group in Gastrointestinal and Abdominal Radiology (SIGGAR); one comparing computed tomographic colonography (CTC) and barium enema (BE),[16] the other CTC and colonoscopy.[17] Each trial had a 2:1 randomisation in favour of the "default" whole-colon examination. Eligible patients were those ≥ 55 years with symptoms or signs suggestive of colorectal cancer who were fit to undergo full bowel preparation, had no known genetic predisposition to cancer, no history of inflammatory bowel disease, no whole-colon examination in the past six months and were not in active follow-up for previous colorectal cancer. The primary outcome measure for the CTC versus colonoscopy trial was the requirement for additional tests needed to diagnose or exclude significant neoplasia. For the CTC versus BE study it was detection rates and diagnostic sensitivity of significant colonic neoplasia by each test.

The results of the first sub-trial[16] demonstrated that CTC detects significantly more colorectal cancers or large polyps than BE (93/1277 7·3% vs 141/2527 5·6%, relative risk 1·31, 95%CI 1·01–1·68; p = ·039) and has a lower miss rate for colorectal cancer (CTC missed three of 45 colorectal cancers and BE missed 12 of 85). Rates of additional colonic investigation were higher after CTC than after BE due to higher detection rates of both large and small polyps. Given that CTC is a less burdensome procedure for patients and affords the opportunity to refer patients for same day colonoscopy, it is likely that it should replace BE in this setting.

Key Point

• CT colonography should be the preferred radiological test over BE for investigation of symptomology suggestive of colorectal cancer.

The results of the other sub-trial,[17] CTC versus colonoscopy, have generated more discussion. In terms of detection rates of colorectal cancer or large polyps there was no difference, 11% for both procedures. CTC missed just one of 29 colorectal cancers and colonoscopy missed none of 55. There was no difference in serious adverse events. CTC did generate substantially more follow-up tests than colonoscopy (30·0% vs 8·2% relative risk 3·65, 95%CI 2·87–4·65; p < ·0001) with almost half of the referrals being for small (<10 mm) polyps of clinical uncertainty. As such there was a low probability of finding cancer or a large polyp on follow-up tests. The authors suggested that many of these follow-up investigations might be avoided by the development of guidelines for patient referral and the use of techniques such as faecal tagging to increase specificity. At present the number of other referrals for incidental findings detected by CT is not reported.

Key Point

• Although CT colonography provides a similarly sensitive and less invasive alternative to colonoscopy, the high referral rates will need to be addressed.

Laparoscopic Surgery for Colorectal Cancer

Two trials were published in 2013 comparing laparoscopic to open resection for colorectal cancer: long-term follow-up of the MRC CLASICC trial,[18] and short-term results of the COLOR II trial.[19] The MRC CLASICC (Conventional versus Laparoscopic-Assisted Surgery in Colorectal Cancer) trial was commenced in 1996. Unlike similar studies launched in other countries this trial was the only one to include rectal cancers and undertake standardised reporting and central review of pathology specimens. The short-term outcomes of the trial, first published in 2005, demonstrated higher, albeit not significantly, rates of positive circumferential resection margin involvement following laparoscopic anterior resection.[20] However, at three-year follow-up there was no difference in terms of local recurrence rates[21] and five-year follow-up data similarly showed no differences in terms of overall survival, disease-free survival or local and distant recurrence between the groups.[22] The long-term results published in 2013, at a median follow-up of 62 months, continue to support the use of laparoscopic surgery for both colonic and rectal cancer.[18] Median overall survival for colonic cancer was 85·1 months and rectal cancer 73·6 months with no statistically significant difference between the groups.

The **CO**lorectal cancer **L**aparoscopic or **O**pen **R**esection (COLOR II) trial compared laparoscopic to open surgery in patients with rectal cancer and was of a non-inferiority design. The short-term results published in early 2013 demonstrated equivalent findings in terms of safety and resection margin.[19] Whilst laparoscopic operations took longer (240 min vs 188 min, $p < ·0001$), there was a lower intraoperative blood loss (median 200 mL vs 400 mL $p < ·0001$). In addition bowel function returned sooner (2·0 days vs 3·0 days, $p < ·0001$) and hospital stay was shorter (8·0 days vs 9·0 days, $p = ·036$) in the laparoscopic group. There was no standardisation of perioperative protocols in this study and notably ERPs were not mandated. The protocol simply stated that within each centre open and laparoscopic patients were to be managed similarly. The length-of-stay figures were better than in the CLASICC trial, although of course the first patients were randomised to the respective studies eight-years apart. As such, it is likely that in COLOR II the majority of centres would have used principles of enhanced recovery. Similarly, the operative conversion rate of 16% in COLOR II, compared to 29% in CLASICC likely reflects the additional experience that has been gained with time.

Key Point

- There is now considerable trial evidence to support the use of laparoscopic surgery for resection of both colonic and rectal cancer.

BREAST

Intraoperative Radiotherapy

Intraoperative radiotherapy (IORT) delivers a high dose of radiation precisely to the targeted area with minimal exposure of surrounding tissues and has been found to be feasible in the management of a number of solid tumours.

The results of two trials, ELIOT[23] and TARGIT-A,[24] examining the role of IORT for women undergoing breast-conserving surgery became available in 2013 and have generated considerable discussion. The use of IORT removes the need to attend a radiotherapy centre daily for up to six weeks, which is stressful and inconvenient meaning that many women worldwide who live remote from such facilities undergo mastectomy. These trials were undertaken to determine whether IORT could be shown to be non-inferior to external beam radiotherapy (EBRT) in reducing local recurrence. Each trial compared a different type of IORT with EBRT, and the primary outcome was recurrence in the conserved breast.

TARGIT-A utilised the Intrabeam device (Carl Zeiss Meditec, Oberkochen, Germany), which provides a point source of 50 kV energy X-rays at the centre of a spherical applicator, whereas ELIOT used linear accelerators to undertake the electron IORT technique. Both were non-inferiority trials; in ELIOT the prespecified equivalence margin was local recurrence of 7·5% in the IORT group and the TARGIT-A trial had a prespecified non-inferiority margin of 2·5% at five years. Overall in TARGIT-A, the five-year risks for local recurrence in the conserved breast for IORT versus whole-breast irradiation were 3·3% (95%CI 2·1–5·1) versus 1·3% (0·7–2·5; $p = ·042$). TARGIT-A did however contain both pre-pathology, with IORT delivered at the time of lumpectomy, and post-pathology strata with IORT delivered as a second procedure by reopening the wound. When just the pre-pathology stratum was considered, that is those patients randomised before lumpectomy, the results were 2·1% (95% CI 1·1–4·2) for IORT and 1·1% (0·5–2·5) for whole breast radiotherapy ($p = ·31$). By contrast ELIOT did not allow a post-pathology procedure. After a median follow-up of 5·8 years in the ELIOT trial, the five-year event rate for IBTR was 4·4% (95%CI 2·7–6·1) with IORT and 0·4% (0·0–1·0) with whole-breast irradiation. Although the event rate is higher in the EBRT group, both trials met their pre-defined criteria to conclude that IORT is non-inferior to EBRT.

Following these trials it is now argued that IORT is an acceptable alternative to EBRT in selected patients.[25,26] Indeed, it may be preferable given that it can be completed in one procedure and in some parts of the world may avoid mastectomy. Others are less convinced with heavy criticism of both trial design and analysis.[27,28] Indeed, some argue that present follow-up is currently too immature to determine whether IORT is sufficiently efficacious to replace EBRT. However, it is clear that the technique warrants evaluation and guidance on the use of the intrabeam radiotherapy system for early breast cancer is currently in development by the National Institute of Health and Care Excellence.

Key Point

- IORT may offer a safe and effective alternative to EBRT in selected patients undergoing breast-conserving surgery.

REFERENCES

1. Obesity: Guidance on the prevention, identification, assessment and management of overweight and obesity in adults and children. NICE guidelines [CG43]. [2006] Available from http://www.nice.org.uk/guidance/CG43. Accessed 6th August 2014.

2. Ikramuddin S, Korner J, Lee WJ, et al. Roux-en-Y gastric bypass vs intensive medical management for the control of type 2 diabetes, hypertension, and hyperlipidemia: the Diabetes Surgery Study randomized clinical trial. JAMA: the journal of the American Medical Association. 2013;309(21):2240-9.

3. Liang Z, Wu Q, Chen B, et al. Effect of laparoscopic Roux-en-Y gastric bypass surgery on type 2 diabetes mellitus with hypertension: a randomized controlled trial. Diabetes Res Clin Pract. 2013;101(1):50-6.

4. Gloy VL, Briel M, Bhatt DL, et al. Bariatric surgery versus non-surgical treatment for obesity: a systematic review and meta-analysis of randomised controlled trials. BMJ. 2013;347:f5934.

5. Grant AM, Cotton SC, Boachie C, et al. Minimal access surgery compared with medical management for gastro-oesophageal reflux disease: five year follow-up of a randomised controlled trial (REFLUX). BMJ. 2013;346:f1908.

6. Jones C, Kelliher L, Dickinson M, et al. Randomized clinical trial on enhanced recovery versus standard care following open liver resection. Br J Surg. 2013;100(8):1015-24.

7. Torgerson DJ, Roberts C. Understanding controlled trials. Randomisation methods: concealment. BMJ. 1999;319(7206):375-6.

8. O'Neill S, Leuschner S, McNally SJ, et al. Meta-analysis of ischaemic preconditioning for liver resections. Br J Surg. 2013;100(13):1689-700.

9. Orci LA, Toso C, Mentha G, et al. Systematic review and meta-analysis of the effect of perioperative steroids on ischaemia-reperfusion injury and surgical stress response in patients undergoing liver resection. Br J Surg. 2013;100(5): 600-9.

10. Topal B, Fieuws S, Aerts R, et al. Pancreaticojejunostomy versus pancreaticogastrostomy reconstruction after pancreaticoduodenectomy for pancreatic or periampullary tumours: a multicentre randomised trial. Lancet Oncol. 2013;14(7):655-62.

11. Figueras J, Sabater L, Planellas P, et al. Randomized clinical trial of pancreaticogastrostomy versus pancreaticojejunostomy on the rate and severity of pancreatic fistula after pancreaticoduodenectomy. Br J Surg. 2013;100(12):1597-605.

12. Wolfgang CL, Pawlik TM. Pancreaticoduodenectomy: time to change our approach? Lancet Oncol. 2013;14(7):573-5.

13. Goh BK. Randomized clinical trial of pancreaticogastrostomy versus pancreaticojejunostomy on the rate and severity of pancreatic fistula after pancreaticoduodenectomy (Br J Surg 2013; 100: 1597-1605). Br J Surg. 2014;101(3):289-90.

14. Trastulli S, Cirocchi R, Desiderio J, et al. Systematic review and meta-analysis of randomized clinical trials comparing single-incision versus conventional laparoscopic cholecystectomy. Br J Surg. 2013;100(2):191-208.

15. Rosenmuller MH, Thoren Ornberg M, Myrnas T, et al. Expertise-based randomized clinical trial of laparoscopic versus small-incision open cholecystectomy. Br J Surg. 2013;100(7):886-94.

16. Halligan S, Wooldrage K, Dadswell E, et al. Computed tomographic colonography versus barium enema for diagnosis of colorectal cancer or large polyps in symptomatic patients (SIGGAR): a multicentre randomised trial. Lancet. 2013;381(9873):1185-93.

17. Atkin W, Dadswell E, Wooldrage K, et al. Computed tomographic colonography versus colonoscopy for investigation of patients with symptoms suggestive of colorectal cancer (SIGGAR): a multicentre randomised trial. Lancet. 2013;381(9873): 1194-202.

18. Green BL, Marshall HC, Collinson F, et al. Long-term follow-up of the Medical Research Council CLASICC trial of conventional versus laparoscopically assisted resection in colorectal cancer. Br J Surg. 2013;100(1):75-82.

19. van der Pas MH, Haglind E, Cuesta MA, et al. Laparoscopic versus open surgery for rectal cancer (COLOR II): short-term outcomes of a randomised, phase 3 trial. Lancet Oncol. 2013;14(3):210-8.

20. Guillou PJ, Quirke P, Thorpe H, et al. Short-term endpoints of conventional versus laparoscopic-assisted surgery in patients with colorectal cancer (MRC CLASICC trial): multicentre, randomised controlled trial. Lancet. 2005;365(9472):1718-26.

21. Jayne DG, Guillou PJ, Thorpe H, et al. Randomized trial of laparoscopic-assisted resection of colorectal carcinoma: 3-year results of the UK MRC CLASICC Trial Group. J Clin Oncol. 2007;25(21):3061-8.

22. Jayne DG, Thorpe HC, Copeland J, et al. Five-year follow-up of the Medical Research Council CLASICC trial of laparoscopically assisted versus open surgery for colorectal cancer. Br J Surg. 2010;97(11):1638-45.

23. Veronesi U, Orecchia R, Maisonneuve P, et al. Intraoperative radiotherapy versus external radiotherapy for early breast cancer (ELIOT): a randomised controlled equivalence trial. Lancet Oncol. 2013;14(13):1269-77.

24. Vaidya JS, Wenz F, Bulsara M, et al. Risk-adapted targeted intraoperative radiotherapy versus whole-breast radiotherapy for breast cancer: 5-year results for local control and overall survival from the TARGIT-A randomised trial. Lancet. 2014;383(9917):603-13.

25. Azria D, Lemanski C. Intraoperative radiotherapy for breast cancer. Lancet. 2014;383(9917):578-81.

26. Vaidya JS, Wenz F, Bulsara M, et al. Radiotherapy for breast cancer, the TARGIT-A trial—Authors' reply. Lancet. 2014;383(9930):1719-20.

27. Haviland JS, A'Hern R, Bentzen SM, et al. Radiotherapy for breast cancer, the TARGIT-A trial. Lancet. 2014;383(9930):1716-7.

28. Cuzick J. Radiotherapy for breast cancer, the TARGIT-A trial. Lancet. 2014;383 (9930):1716.

Index

Page numbers followed by *t* refer to table, *f* refer to figure and *fc* refer to flow chart.

A

Abiraterone 141
Abscess, perianal 108
Adenocanthoma of
  pancreatic head 92
  stomach 55, 56
  pancreatic 91, 93
ADT 131, 138
  side effects of 141
Advanced airway skills 26
Advanced trauma life support
    course 12
Adverse events 15
Albumin 39, 46
  interstitial 39
  plasma 39
Aldosterone 39, 40
Alpha-fetoprotein 57
Anaemia
  iron deficiency 57*t*
  pernicious 56*t*
Anaesthesia
  epidural 104
  intravenous 104
  spinal single shot 104
Anaesthesia induced hypovolaemia
    39, 46
Anaesthesia induced vasodilatation 39
Anal canal 109, 111
Anal fistula
  advanced treatments 111
  classification 110
  clinical examination of patient
    in 109
  complex, treatment 111
  Crohn's 108, 109, 112, 113*t*, 114*t*
  cryptoglandular 108, 112, 113*t*, 114*t*
  diagnosis 108
  endo-anal ultrasonography in 109
  faecal incontinence risk 110
  high 110
  imaging in 109
  in carcinoma 108
  in HIV 108
  in tuberculosis 108
  intersphincteric 110
  laser closure 117
  low 110
  magnetic resonance imaging in 109
  pathogenesis 108
  primary 108
  simple 111
  tract 110
  tract filling 111*fc*, 112
    anal fistula plug 112
    glues 112
  tract ligation 111*fc*, 115
  tract obliteration 111*fc*, 116
  trans-sphincteric 110
Anal sepsis 108
Anal sphincter
  external 109, 110
  internal 109
  muscles 111
Androgen Deprivation Therapy
    See ADT
Anorectal advancement flap 115
Anorectal junction 109
Anthracycline, in gastric cancer
    metastatis 67
Anti-diuretic hormone 39, 104
Anti-EGFR monoclonal antibodies, in
    colorectal cancer 163, 164
Anti-reflux barrier 76
Anti-reflux surgery 74, 75, 80
  complications 77
  failure of 79
  outcomes 77
  persistent symptoms 80
  type I failures 80
  type II failures 80
  type III failures 80
Anti-TNF agents 109
  in Crohn's anal fistula 117
Aortic aneurysm surgery 19
Aquamantys system 165
ARO 96-02 138

Arterial resection, in pancreatic
    cancer 93
Artery, hepatic 88
Axillary lymphadenopathy, in phyllodes
    tumour 148
Azzopardi and Salvadori criteria,
    diagnosis of phyllodes tumour
    nature 150*t*

B

Bariatric surgery 19, 193, 194
Barium enema 197
Barium radiographs, in GORD 73
Barrett's intestinal metaplasia 72
Barrett's oesophagus 73, 75
Basic colonoscopy courses 13
Bevacizumab, in colorectal
    cancer 163, 164
Body mass index (BMI) 193
Bowel preparation 102, 103
Bowel resection 101
Brachytherapy, for prostate cancer
    136, 138
Bravo telemetry system 74
Breast
    conserving surgery 153
    hamartomas 147
    intraoperative radiotherapy 199
    prosthesis 153
    reconstruction 153, 157
Cabazitaxel 142
Calcium 40, 47
Calf muscle-pump failure 175
Cancer
    breast 61
    colorectal 160
        extra-hepatic metastases 168
        laparoscopic surgery for 198
    gastric 55, 64
        adjuvant chemoradiation therapy
            in 64
        alarm features 57*t*
        classification of 55
        complete surgical resection 59
        computed tomography (CT) 58
        diagnosis of 57
        endoscopic resection 59
        endoscopic ultrasound 58
        HER2-positive 66
        laparoscopy peritoneal
            washings 58

    risk factors associated 56*t*
    staging of 59*t*
    treatment 58
oesophageal 64, 72
oesophagogastric junction 64
pancreatic 87
    AHPBA/ SSO/ SSAT
        classification 88, 90
    borderline resectable 88, 89, 90
    MDACC classification 88, 90
    neo-adjuvant oncological
        treatment 91
    NCCN criteria 89
    resectable 89
    unresectable 89, 90
    venous resection 92
prostate 131
    diagnosis 132
    metastatic disease 140
    natural history of 135
    treatment 135
rectal 123
    laparoscopic surgery 124
    robotic surgery 124

C

Capecitabine, for metastatic gastric
    cancer 67
Carbohydrate antigen 57
Carcinoid tumours, of stomach 56
Cardiomyotomy, for achalasia 76
Cardiovascular disease, due to ADT 141
Care of critically ill surgical patient 12
Case-based discussions 6
Catheters
    arterial line 104
    central venous 104
CCRISP *See* Care of the critically ill
    surgical patient
Cetuximab, in colorectal cancer 163
Chloride 41, 45-47, 49
Cholecystectomy 196
Cisplatin, for metastatic gastric
    cancer 67
CLASICC trial 199
Clinical encounters 6
Colectomy, total 126
Collis gastroplasty 80
Colloids 46
Colonic investigations 197
Colonoscopy 197, 198

Color II trial 198
Colorectal resection 106
Colorectal surgery
    incision
        infra-umbilical 105
        modified pfannenstiel 105
        transverse 105
    laparoscopic 101
    robotic 120-127
Combat applicator tourniquet 29*f*
Compression, varicose veins 183
Computed tomographic colonoscopy
    197, 198
Confidential air human factors incident
    reporting programme 16
Confidential enquiry into
    maternal and child health 21
    suicide and homicide 21
Confidential reporting 15, 23
Confidential reporting system for
    surgery 16, 17, 18, 19
CORESS *See* Confidential reporting
    system for surgery
CORESS lite 18
CORESS process 18*fc*
Cortisol 39
CRITICS trial 66
Crohn's disease 108
Cryotherapy for
    prostate cancer 139
    prostate cancer, side effects 140
Crystalloids 46, 48
CTC *See* Computed tomographic
    colonoscopy
Cystosarcoma phyllodes 147

D

dA Vinci robots 124, 126
dA Vinci robots Xi 127
Damage control resuscitation (DCR) 26
Deep perforators 175
Deep venous thrombosis 175
Diabetes, due to ADT 141
Diabetes surgery study 193
Direct observation of procedural
    skills 6
Diverticula, in oesophagus 74
Downsizing chemotherapy, in SCLM
    161
DP-CAR 93
Duodenogastric reflux 75

Duplex USS imaging, for Venus
    reflux 177
Dysphagia in 72
    fundoplication 77-79
    gastric cancer 57

E

Edinburgh vein study 175
Electrolyte assessment, in surgery 42
Endocinch procedure 82
Endoscopic mucosal resection, in
    gastric cancer 63
Endoscopic submucosal dissection,
    in gastric cancer 63
Endoscopic suturing 82
Endoscopy, in GORD 73
EndoStim LES stimulation system 83
Endothermal ablation, in venus
    reflux 178
Endovascular aneurysm repair
    procedures 12
Endovenous laser ablation, in venus
    reflux 179
Endovenous techniques, venus
    reflux 178
Enhanced recovery after surgery,
    principles of 102*f*
Enhanced recovery pathways
    (ERPS) 194
Enhanced recovery programme 101
    perioperative
        care 103
        interventions 101
    postoperative
        care 101
        fluid replacement 105
        high concentrations of
            electrolytes 105
        interventions 105
    preoperative interventions 101, 102
Enzalutamide 141
EORTC 22911 138
EORTC 40983 163, 164
Epstein criteria 136
Erectile dysfunction, in prostate cancer
    treatment 139
ERP *See* Enhanced recovery
    programme
ERSPC *See* European randomized study
    of screening for prostate cancer
ESCHAR study 183

Esophyx procedure 82
ESPAC-5 trial 91
European randomized study of
    screening for prostate
    cancer 131, 132
European working time directive 10
EVLA, in venus reflux 181
Extended oesophageal dissection 77
External beam radiotherapy, for
    prostate cancer 136

F

Fibroadenoma, breast 147, 154*fc*
Fibroepithelial tumour, of breast 147
FILAC 117
Fistula-in-ano *See* anal fistula
Fistulotomy 109, 110, 111
Fluid loss, abnormal 49*f*
Fluid resuscitation 44*fc*, 43
    colloids 45
    crystalloids 45
    human albumin 45
Fluoropyrimidine doublet, in metastatic
    gastric cancer 67
Folfox chemotherapy, in SCLM 163, 164
Fundoplication
    endoscopic 82
    failures 80
    Nissen 76
    partial 77
        anterior 76
        posterior 76
    side effects of 77
    slipped 80
    total 77

G

Gas-bloat, in Nissen fundoplication 76
Gastrectomy 60
    laparoscopic 63
    radical 59
    subtotal 59
    total 59
Gastric banding 193
Gastric cancer, chemotherapy in 64
Gastric perforation, during anti-reflux
    surgery 79
Gastritis, atrophic 73
Gastro-oesophageal

junction 57, 72
    tumours 57
Gastro-oesophageal reflux
    disease 72, 194
Gelatins 46
General surgery curriculum 4, 5*t*
    advanced trauma surgery 5*t*
    bariatric 5*t*
    benign upper GI 5*t*
    breast surgery 5*t*
    colorectal surgery 5*t*
    emergency surgery 5*t*
    endocrine surgery 5*t*
    functional colorectal surgery 5*t*
    general surgery of childhood 5*t*
    hepatobiliary 5*t*
    hepatopancreatobiliary 5*t*
    oesophagogastric 5*t*
    pancreatic 5*t*
    pelvic floor surgery 5*t*
    remote and rural surgery 5*t*
    transplant surgery 5*t*
GI bleeding
    lower 57*t*
    upper 57*t*
GI dysfunction, postoperative 43
Glucagon-like peptide-1 agonist 193
Glucose, intravenous 40, 47, 48
GOJ *See* Gastro-oesophageal junction
GORD *See* Gastro-oesophageal reflux
    disease
Gynaecomastia, due to ADT 141

H

H2 receptor antagonists 73
Haematemesis 57
Haemorrhage
    (C) atastrophic 27
    massive 31*fc*
Hand-held Doppler, for venus
    reflux 177
Hartmann's solution 46
HBA1C 193
HDAC1 *See* Histone deacetylase 1
Healthcare quality improvement
    programme (HQIP) 20
Helicobacter pylori 56, 56*t*
Hemicolectomy, right 123
Hepatectomies
    in SCLM 166
    Two-stage, in SCLM 161

Hepatic resections, in SCLM 165
Hiatal repair 77
Hiatus hernias 74-76
HIFU *See* High-intensity focused
    ultrasound
High-intensity focused ultrasound
    for prostate cancer 136, 139
    side effects 140
Histone deacetylase 1 151
Hydroxyethyl starch 46
Hyperchloraemia 41, 50
Hyperchloraemic acidosis 41
Hyperkalaemia 40, 44*fc*, 50
Hypertension, superficial venous 175
Hypochloraemic alkalosis 41
Hypokalaemia 40, 44*fc*
Hypokalaemic alkalosis 40
Hyponatraemia 41, 44*fc*
    dilutional 40
    postoperative 40
Hypotension
    due to epidurals 104
    postoperative 104
Hypothalamic–pituitary–gonadal
    axis 140
Hypothalamus 140

I

IAT *See* Intermittent androgen therapy
Incident report form 22*f*
Inflammatory bowel disease 197
Insulin resistance, postoperative 102
Intensity modulated radiotherapy, for
    prostate cancer 137
Intercollegiate surgical curriculum
    project 4
Intermittent androgen therapy 141
Intersphincteric fistula tract, ligation
    of 115
Intra-hepatic veno-occlusive
    disease 165
Intraperitoneal therapy, in gastric
    cancer 66
Intravenous fluid therapy in surgery
    4R approach 43
    5th reassessment 45
    assessment of 42
    National Institute for Health and Care
        Excellence, algorithms 44*fc*
    National Institute for Health and Care
        Excellence, training tool 39

Irinotecan in
    colorectal cancer 163
    SCLM 164
Ischaemia reperfusion injury 195

J

Jaundice 57*t*
Joint committee on surgical training 11
Journal of hand surgery 18
JVP 43

L

Laparoscopic revisional surgery, after
    anti-reflux surgery 80
Laryngitis 72
LDL cholesterol 193
Left ventricular mass index 193
Lethal triad of trauma 30
Levator plate 109
Likert scale 134
Linitis plastica 56
Linx reflux system 83
Liver injury, during anti-reflux
    surgery 79
Luteinizing hormone 140
Lymph node
    axillary, in phyllodes tumour 153
    gastric 62*t*
Lymphadenectomy
    in gastric cancer 60
        D1 60, 61, 64
        D2 60, 61
        D3 61
Lymphoma 55

M

Magnesium 40, 41, 47
Malignancy, intra-abdominal 175
Malnutrition, postoperative 40
Manometry 74
Mastectomy 155
    in phyllodes tumour 155
Medical training application service 7
Medigus SRS procedure 82
Melaena 57
Metachronous colorectal liver
    metastases 160, 161
Modernising medical careers
    initiative 3

Molecular therapy
   breast 66
   colorectal 66
   lung cancers 66
MPMRI *See* Multiparametric MRI
MRC clasicc trial 198
Multiparametric MRI, for prostate
     biopsy 133, 134
Multi-source feedback (MSF) 6
Muscle
   anal 108
   rectal 126

N

Nasogastric drainage 104
National clinical assessment service 21
National confidential enquiry into
    patient outcomes and
      deaths 19, 20
National confidential enquiry into
    perioperative deaths 19
National health service 15, 19, 21, 22,
   23, 25
National institute for health and care
    excellence 38
National reporting and learning
    service 19, 21, 23
NDO plicator 82
Nerves, hypogastric 126
Nice guidelines, on nutrition
    support 41
Nitrogen balance, postoperative 102
NO16966 trial 164
Nontechnical skills for surgeons 12
Non-thermal ablative methods 180
NPSA 21, 23

O

Oesophageal high definition
    manometry 80
Oesophageal impedance measurement
   74
Oesophageal motility disorders 74
Oesophageal sphincter, lower 72
Oesophagitis 73
Oliguria, postoperative 40
Opiates, long-acting 105
Orchidectomy, bilateral, in prostate
    cancer 140
Organ dysfunction, postoperative 42
Orthopaedic surgery, computer-assisted
   12

Oxaliplatin in
   colorectal cancer 163
   metastatic gastric cancer 67
   SCLM 164

P

Paddington clinicopathological
    suspicious score 150
Pancreatectomy 60, 68, 92
   distal 93
Pancreatic anastomosis 195
Pancreatic drain 49*f*
Pancreaticoduodenectomy 91, 195
Panitumumab, in colorectal cancer 163
Paraoesophageal hiatus herniation 77
Parietal cell hyperplasia 73
Parks' classification 110
Patient safety incident report from 22*f*
PDVR 92
Pelvic vein reflux 184
Penetrating trauma 25
Pharyngitis 72
Phosphate 40
Phyllodes tumour 147
   benign 149, 150, 154*fc*
     recurrence of 155
   borderline 154*fc*, 155
   clinical presentation 147
   core needle biopsy 150
   fine-needle aspiration cytology 149
   high-resolution ultrasound 148
   immunohistochemistry 151
   lung parenchyma involvement 155
   magnetic resonance imaging 149
   malignant 149, 150, 152, 154*fc*,155
   mammography 148
   management of 152, 154*fc*
   mastectomy 153
   metastasis 155
     bone 155
     heart 155
     liver 155
     lungs 155
   metastatic 156*fc*
   molecular analysis 151
   recurrence 155
     management of 156*fc*
   role of pathological analysis 149
Pituitary, anterior 140
Platinum, in metastatic gastric
    cancer 67

Pneumothorax, during anti-reflux
    surgery 79
Polidocanol, in sclerotherapy 179
Portal superior mesenteric vein
    resection 92
Portal vein resection 91
Portal venous embolisation, in
    SCLM 161
Potassium 40
    depletion, postoperative 40
Procedure-based assessments 6
Prostate, lung, colorectal and ovarian
    cancer screening trial 132
Prostatectomy
    radical 132, 136, 137
       retropubic 134
       robotic 138*f*
Prostate-specific antigen *See* PSA
Proton-pump inhibitors (PPIs) 73
PSA 131, 132, 136, 141
    doubling time 136
    screening 131
       American Urological
          Association 132
       British Association of Urological
          surgeons 132
       ERSPC 132
       PLCO 132
       United States preventative
          services task force 132
PT *See* Phyllodes tumour

R

Radiofrequency ablation in
    SCLM 161
    venus reflux 179
Radiotherapy and oncology
    group scale 140
Radiotherapy, in gastric cancer 64
RAS homolog enriched in brain 151
REACTIVE trial 181
Rectal cancer resections, in SCLM 166
Rectal prolapse
    external 126
    internal 126
Recurrent varices after surgery 185
Redistribution, of intravenous fluid 43,
    44*fc*, 48
Refeeding syndrome 41
Reflux questionnaire 194

Reflux trial 194
Renin–angiotensin 39
Renin–angiotensin-aldosterone
    pathways 104
Replacement, of intravenous fluid 43,
    44*fc*, 48
Resuscitation, after trauma 30
Resuscitative thoracotomy 26
REVAS *See* Recurrent varices after
    surgery
RFA *See* Radiofrequency ablation
RHEB *See* Ras homolog enriched in
    brain
Ringer's lactate/acetate 46
Rings, in oesophagus 74
Robotic assisted, kidney transplant 120
Robotic colorectal surgery, anterior
    resection 123
Robotic radical prostatectomy 120, 121
Robotic surgery 120
    advantages 120
    beating heart coronary artery bypass
       graft 120
    cholecystectomy 120
    disadvantages 120
    fallopian tube reconnection 120
    in gastric cancer 64
    single access 27 multi-quadrant 127
Robotic technique
    mesorectal excision 124
    pelvic nerve damage 124
ROLARR 124
Routine maintenance, of intravenous
    fluid 43, 44*fc*
    best regimen for 47
Roux-En-Y gastric bypass surgery 193
Royal London code red protocol 31*fc*
Royal Marsden criteria 136
RTOG *See* Radiotherapy and oncology
    group scale

S

Sacrocolporectopexy, laparoscopic 126
Safety alerts 21
Saphenofemoral junction 175
Saphenopopliteal junction 175
Scandinavian prostate cancer group-4
    trial 135
Sclerotherapy
    in venus reflux 179

benefits 180
complications 180
mechano chemical ablation 180
steam ablation 180
SCLM *See* Synchronous colorectal liver
metastases
Sentinel lymph node biopsy 61
Sinusoidal injury 165
Sister Mary Joseph's nodule 57
Sleeve gastrectomy 193
Small incision open cholecystectomy
197
Sodium 39, 40
Sodium chloride solution, intravenous
41, 46-48, 50
Sodium tetradecyl sulphate 179
SOLARR 124
SPCG-4 Scandinavian prostate cancer
group-4 trial
Splenectomy 60, 68
Splenopancreatectomy 60
Squamous cell carcinoma, of
stomach 56
Stab wound 25
cardiac tamponade 26
catastrophic haemorrhage 26
tension pneumothorax 26
Starling's curve 104
Steatohepatitis
alcoholic 164
non-alcoholic 164
Stretta procedure 82
Stromal tumours, of stomach 56
Superior mesenteric vein occlusion 88
Surgical curriculum 12
Surgical mishaps 15
Surgical simulation 11
Surgical specialties, selection into 7
Surgical training
assessment in 5
curricula in 3
within modern working
regulations 10
SWOG 8794 138
Synchronous colorectal liver metastases
160, 161, 166
18F-FDG PET/CT 161
chemotherapy 163
computed tomography (CT) 161
gadoxetic acid enhanced and
diffusion-weighted MRI 161

irresectable 167
adjunctive treatments 168
defunctioning colostomy 168
hepatic arterial infusion with
chemotherapy 168
laser recanalisation 168
primary tumour resection 168
stenting 168
stereotactic body radiotherapy
168
liver-first approach 160
management of 162*fc*
radiological evaluation 161, 162*fc*

T

Tap test 177
Temple report 10
Testosterone 140, 141
Thoracostomy
bilateral 28
unilateral 28
Thrombophlebitis, due to RFA in venus
reflux 181
Tranexamic acid, pre-hospital use 26
Transanalsurgery 126
Transperineal biopsies, for prostate
biopsy 133
Transrectal ultrasound-guided biopsies,
for prostate cancer 132
Trauma management 26
Trendelenburg position, for colorectal
procedures 121
TRUS biopsies 134

U

USS-guided FS, for venous reflux 181

V

VAAFT, in anal fistula 117
Varicose veins 175, 176*t*, 177
surgery, recurrence 184
Varicosities
primary 175
secondary 175
Vascular society 18
Vein
femoral 177
long saphenous 175, 177

SFJ flush ligation 178
stripping of 178
portal 88
occlusion 88
superior mesenteric 88
Venous disease, lower CEAP
(clinical, etiology, anatomy,
pathophysiology) classification
of 176*t*
Venous reflux 175, 177
open surgery 177

Venous ulceration 181
Ventral mesh rectopexy 125
for internal rectal prolapse 126
laparoscopic 126
Virchow's node 57

W

Waldeyer's fascia 126
WEE1 homolog 151
Workplace-based assessments 6